D0017085

The Ultimate
BICYCLE OWNER'S
MANUAL

The Ultimate BICYCLE OWNER'S MANUAL

The Universal Guide to Bikes, Riding, and Everything for Beginner and Seasoned Cyclists

|||||||||||||||||||||||||||||||||

EBEN WEISS

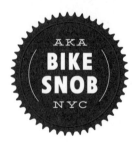

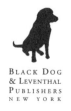

BLACK DOG
& LEVENTHAL
PUBLISHERS
NEW YORK

Black Dog & Leventhal Publishers
Hachette Book Group / 1290 Avenue of the Americas / New York, NY 10104
www.blackdogandleventhal.com

Printed in the United States of America

RRD-C

First edition: May 2016

10 9 8 7 6 5 4 3 2 1

Black Dog & Leventhal Publishers is an imprint of Hachette Books, a division of
Hachette Book Group.

The Black Dog & Leventhal Publishers name and logo are trademarks of Hachette
Book Group, Inc.

The publisher is not responsible for websites (or their content) that are not owned
by the publisher.

Library of Congress Cataloging-in-Publication Data
Names: Weiss, Eben, author.
Title: The ultimate bicycle owner's manual : the universal guide to bikes, riding,
and everything for beginner and seasoned cyclists / Eben Weiss.
Description: First edition. | New York : Black Dog & Leventhal, 2016. |
    Includes index.
Identifiers: LCCN 2015041449| ISBN 9780316352680 (paperback) | ISBN
    9780316352673 (ebook)
Subjects: LCSH: Cycling—Handbooks, manuals, etc. | Bicycles--Maintenance and
    repair—Handbooks, manuals, etc. | BISAC: SPORTS & RECREATION / Cycling. |
    SPORTS & RECREATION / Reference. | HEALTH & FITNESS / Exercise.
Classification: LCC GV1041 .W454 2016 | DDC 796.6—dc23 LC record available
    at http://lccn.loc.gov/2015041449

To everyone who is about
to discover the joy, beauty, and
practicality of cycling.

Contents

Chapter 1

OBTAINING A BIKE

S o you've decided to get a bicycle.
Congratulations!
If you feel confused and overwhelmed by the vast and bewildering bicycle marketplace, don't worry, because admitting you need help is the first step toward becoming a cyclist. Before we go any further, it will help if you have a basic understanding of the history of the bicycle.

IN THE BEGINNING

In the 1870s, buying a bicycle was easy: You went to Ye Olde Velocipede Shoppe, picked out a nice high-wheeler—known as the "penny farthing"—and maybe took a header into a pile of horse manure on the way home. Done. Shopping was easy. The hardest part was riding the thing. First, in order to get started, you had to give the bike a push from behind. Then you had to scramble on top of it while it was rolling, which would have been like climbing onto the roof of a Volkswagen Beetle. Once you were up there, you had to stay up there, which was not easy, thanks to the fact that you were essentially sitting on top of a giant wheel. It's hard to stay upright on a bicycle when your center of gravity is way up on the third floor. If you were able to mount and ride the bike successfully, you still had to climb back down when the ride was over.

Seems like a lot of work, right? Why was that front wheel so gigantic anyway?

Because the penny farthing was propelled by means of a "direct drive," which means the pedals and cranks were attached directly to the front wheel. So, the diameter of the wheel is what determined how fast and far the bicycle would go when your legs turned the pedals. If the wheel was small, you'd have to pedal frantically in order to get anywhere. (Think about how long it would take you to travel a mile on a child's tricycle and you've got the idea.) Therefore, the front wheel was laughably huge.

Even so, people went crazy for the penny farthing, and the world experienced the very first bike boom.

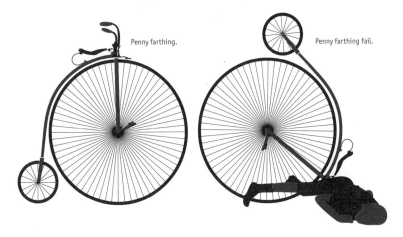

Penny farthing.

Penny farthing fail.

Then, two big things happened.

The Two Big Things

1. In 1885, John Kemp Starley began manufacturing a rear-wheel, chain-drive bicycle with more or less symmetrical wheels.
2. John Boyd Dunlop founded the Dunlop Pneumatic Tire Co. in 1889.

Equal-size wheels? Air-filled tires? This was cycling's chocolate-in-the-peanut-butter moment. Fitting a bicycle with a chain drive meant that you no longer had to change the wheel's diameter in order to optimize the system's mechanical advantage. Instead, the *gear ratio* was determined by the size of the chainring and cogs, which were mounted on the hub of the rear wheel. And presto, a rear-wheel-driven bicycle that could be designed for comfort. Starley's bike, with its diamond frame and two symmetrical wheels, was vastly more stable than a penny farthing, and it was far easier to straddle and ride. As you can imagine, riding a bicycle with symmetrical wheels wrapped in cushions of air was a much more attractive proposition than bouncing around high above the manure-strewn streets on solid tires. It was also a lot safer, for the simple reason that you were much less likely to fall off your bike. In fact, this new design was marketed as the "safety bicycle." By the end of the nineteenth century, pretty much all bicycles were rear-wheel-driven safety bicycles rolling on pneumatic tires. The machine became so popular that cities and municipalities began paving the roads with macadam in order to accommodate the growing legions of cyclists.

So you can thank bicycles for paved roads, and you can also feel free to tell any impatient driver who says "roads are for cars" that they should be thanking *you* for the pavement they're driving on.

TODAY

Now we're well into the twenty-first century, and here you are looking for a bike. The good news is that fundamentally not much has changed about the bicycle since the turn of the last century: We're still (mostly) riding diamond-framed safety bicycles with pneumatic tires. (Yes, there are recumbents and other rethinkings of the upright bicycle, but we'll address those later.) Sure, bikes have gotten a lot lighter, and yes they have much more sophisticated gear changing and braking systems, but if a late nineteenth-century cyclist were to ride through a time wormhole into today, he or she would have no difficulty riding any of my bikes. (Apart from dodging all the cars of course, but we'll address that later as well.)

The bad news is that a century of constant refinement, endless marketing, and incessant hyperspecialization means that shopping for a bicycle can be as vexing as trying to see the UFO in one of those Magic Eye paintings. In fact, you may be so frustrated you're ready to say, "Screw it, I'm leasing a Hyundai." Don't give up. The problem is more with the twenty-first century than it is with cycling. Bikes are simple machines, and unfortunately the simpler something is, the easier it is to ascribe all sorts of mystical attributes to it. That's why people take classes in order to learn how to drink wine, but when they go to lease a Hyundai they'll make their decision based on the location of the cup holder.

DOS AND DON'TS OF CHOOSING A BICYCLE

Ultimately, the secret to choosing a bicycle is avoiding confusion, so here are some basic dos and don'ts to keep you on track, starting with the don'ts.

Don't . . .
✗ ASK ADVICE FROM YOUR NEIGHBOR, ACQUAINTANCE, OR COWORKER WHO RIDES A LOT

First of all, no matter how good-natured this person may seem to be, every cyclist thinks they know everything. Because of this, they're vexed by the notion that they could possibly pour their ocean of knowledge into the tiny, thimble-like vessel that is your brain.

Second, although they *think* they know everything, what they *actually* know pertains only to themselves and their experience. Ask, say, a competitive cyclist what kind of bike you should get, and you'll find yourself on the receiving end of a lecture about frame materials and rotating wheel weight that will make you want to puncture your own eardrums. Eventually you'll find yourself either backing away while nodding politely or simply asleep on your desk in a puddle of your own drool.

Talking to a cyclist is like Coleridge's *The Rime of the Ancient*

Mariner. Any answer from a cyclist starts at the beginning of time, and unless you hit them in the head, it won't end until the sun implodes.

✗ CONSULT THE INTERNET

The Internet is useful for finding pictures of bikes, prices of bikes, locations of bike shops, and even gathering basic information about the pros and cons of various types of bicycles, but for the love of [insert your favorite deity here] *do not engage anybody on it!* At least your competitive cyclist coworker is only one person. When you ask the Internet for advice, you'll get the opinions of one person times a million. When it comes to opinions on bikes, consulting the Internet is learning in a vacuum of stupidity.

✗ CONSULT GLOSSY CYCLING MAGAZINES

"Okay, so the Internet's a great big open source of cluelessness," you're thinking to yourself. "I'll stick to good old-fashioned print. It has integrity."

Sadly, this is not true. Haven't you heard? Print is dead. That's why magazines that are still alive are more beholden than ever to their advertisers for survival. I'm not saying this is a bad thing; magazines contain interesting stories and pretty pictures, and it's advertiser dollars that make this possible. After all, writers don't work for free (though it can sure feel like it).

I'm just saying, never trust a gear review in a magazine (or an online magazine for that matter). Enjoy it, but don't trust it. It's like believing a climate change study funded by the energy lobby.

Do . . .

✔ ADOPT IF POSSIBLE

Bikes are like pets. A fancy purebred might cost you a fortune. Moreover, if you make a decision to purchase one based purely on aesthetics or cachet, that fancy purebred can wind up being a huge and costly mistake. That border collie seemed like a great idea, until you find out that if you don't give it sheep to herd it will dig its way through your living room floor and into the basement. Similarly, that shiny new road bike may capture your fancy, but what happens when you realize you can't carry anything on it and your crotch is numb for six hours after riding it?

It's precisely because so many people make this rookie mistake when buying their first bike that so many countless bikes have been cast aside and are in desperate need of a home. More often than not, you can pick up a cast-off bike for free or close to it.

Talk with friends and neighbors. Check with your building superintendent to see if there are any abandoned bikes in the bike room. Ask your aunt and uncle if that mountain bike your cousin never rode is still sitting in the garage. It may not be perfect. In fact, it may be an utter hunk of crap, but spending no money on crap is a lot better than spending a lot of money on a bike that turns out not to be right for you, and that you in turn wind up abandoning.

Once you find a bike, it's important to *ride it*. It won't take you long to figure out what's right and what's wrong with it. You may be able to change it into the right bike for you just by swapping some parts, or at the very least you'll realize what kind of bike you do need so that when you do go to purchase a brand-new bike, you can spend your money effectively.

Most important, don't get too hung up on how the bike looks. The only way to look good on a bike is to learn how to ride it well.

✔ SHOP FOR A BIKE SHOP, NOT A BIKE

If you're either unable or disinclined to scrounge up a hand-me-down, then, by all means, go to a bike shop. In fact, you'd think if you're looking for a bike that "go to a bike shop" would be the first step on the list, but it's not that simple anymore. First, there are so many different kinds of bike shops now (we'll go into the different kinds in a bit), that it's hard to know where to begin, which can make you just want to give up before you even try. Second, prices at bike shops can be intimidating. Sticker shock may tempt you to shop online instead. Don't. Finding a bike shop you can trust and rely on, and building a relationship with the people who work there, is as important as finding a bike you love to ride.

Pick a few shops in your area, take a deep breath, and go inside. Look around. Strike up a conversation. If you get a good feeling from the staff at one of them, let them sell you a bike. Don't get hung up on whether you can get a slightly better price elsewhere or if the place across town will throw in the upgraded SL Wonk-tronik shifting system for the same price. *None of this matters.* What matters is how well you get along with the shop and its staff, because that's where you're going to be going when the SL Wonk-tronik shifting system starts getting balky.

The bike is almost immaterial, whereas the right bike shop can be the foundation for your entire cycling life ahead.

✔ PULL THE TRIGGER ALREADY

You're not getting married. You're not having a kid. You're not taking out a mortgage on the house where you're going to spend the next fifty years of your life. You're buying a freaking bicycle. Chances are that if it's your first, you're going to want a different one next year. That's okay. Don't shop yourself into a state of indecision or paralysis. Just get a bike between your legs and start riding.

STYLES OF BIKES

Bike companies come up with new types of bicycles as quickly as people figure out new places and ways to ride them. Some bikes go out of style, others come back in. Still others are just old bikes with a new name and a flashy set of decals.

Let's start with the road bikes.

Road Bikes

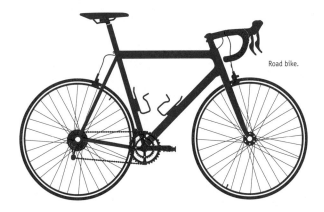

Road bike.

You know those riders who float effortlessly along like they're one with their machines, their immaculate drivetrains whirring like whisks in batter?

Those riders are on road bikes.

You know those riders with the big grease smudges on their calves who careen along the bike path yelling "On your left!" and then fall over at the stoplight because they can't extricate their special shoes from their special pedals?

Those riders are also on road bikes.

No bicycle can be wielded as deftly or as awkwardly as a road bike. It's like a high-quality chef's knife: In the right hands, it's making sushi; in the wrong hands, it's making sushi out of fingers.

So what makes a road bike a road bike? The obvious characteristic is the "drop" handlebars, the primary purpose of which is to allow you to position your body for speed. Riding with your hands in the drops lets you get flat-backed and aero, though many road bike owners lack the flexibility necessary to do this, which leaves them looking like a cabbie at a tollbooth rooting around under the seat for loose change.

Road bikes also tend to have narrow tires for aerodynamics and minimal rolling resistance, as well as saddles that aren't so

Good things about road bikes

- You probably live on or near a road, which means you'll get plenty of use out of your road bike.

- They're more or less the default sporting bicycle, so it's unlikely you're going to come across a shop that doesn't understand them.

- Deal$! The used marketplace is full of used road bike stuff, which means lots of bargains for you.

- They're fairly versatile and designed to be ridden all day so long trips are no problem. Yet with some modifications they're perfect for city use. (You might not want to carry your dog on one, but there's no reason you can't use it to get to work or to the bar.)

- They're responsive machines, and therefore they will teach you a lot about riding. If you can handle a road bike in a variety of situations, you can handle pretty much any type of bike. If you're interested in recreational cycling and you can have only one bike, it should be a road bike.

- They're light and minimal, and while this is mainly to enhance performance, it's also practical for the apartment dweller who has to schlep a bike up and down stairs or store it in the foyer. (Assuming you're one of those Rockefeller types who can afford an apartment with a foyer.)

Bad things about road bikes

- They are not "comfortable," at least in the sense that your TV-watching sweatpants are comfortable. Riding one means "assuming the position," which may not be ideal for those quick jaunts to the store.

- There's a limit to their versatility, which you will discover if you need to carry heavy loads on your bike.

- They're relatively easy to pilfer or steal. You can dismantle a road bike in minutes using about three tools, all of which can fit on a keychain. This is great for a race team mechanic, but not so great for you when you emerge from the shop to find that your handlebars, saddle, and both wheels have been stolen.

much for supporting your body weight as for gently reminding you where to position your posterior. You don't really *sit* on a road bike saddle so much as you lean on it, as you would upon a rattan bench you suspect might give way. In fact, the key to riding a road bike is to distribute your weight evenly across it. If you're doing it

Myths about road bikes

"They're delicate."

This is not true. Road bikes are built to withstand the punishing torque and tube-twisting wattage generated by some of the most powerful athletes on Earth. Sure, in practice they're mostly subjected to the saddle-crushing weight of sedentary Americans who have taken up road cycling as part of a midlife crisis, but they're generally sturdy machines just the same.

"They're not versatile."

Attempting to ride a downhill mountain biking course on a road bike is going to destroy the wheels, possibly the frame, and certainly most of the bones in your skeleton, but extreme use aside, you can do lots of stuff on a road bike. You can even ride them on dirt trails, despite the name "road bike." Although most bike companies would rather sell you another bike specifically for this purpose, you don't need that. Road bikes work well in both town and country, and if you want to put on a pair of flat bars and turn it into a more casual cruising machine, there's nothing stopping you from doing so.

"They're expensive."

Road bikes have never been more expensive, but they've also never been cheaper.

Strictly speaking, road bikes aren't expensive. The truth is they *can* be expensive, and absurdly so. Thanks to carbon fiber, electronics, clever cobranding, and the fickle whims of the 1 percent, road bike manufacturers are managing to tickle the undercarriage of the $20,000 barrier.

At the same time, though, you can buy a perfectly decent road bike for under $1,000.

Best of all, a bike depreciates in value the moment it gets straddled, which means the fickle whims of the 1 percent often become the deep discounts of the 99 percent once the original owner gets bored and moves on to golf or wingsuit flying.

right, you're sort of splayed out on top of it like someone trying to crawl across a frozen pond without falling through the ice.

If all of this sounds wildly impractical, that's because it is, but if your primary reason for wanting a bike is pleasure and speed and not utility, a road bike is a good place to start. Here's why.

ROADS ARE EVERYWHERE

A bike's no good if you don't have somewhere to ride it, and unless you live in a hut in the rainforest you've probably got access to a road of some kind. Even if that road isn't paved, you can still probably ride your road bike on it. In most cases, all you really need to do is change the tires.

ROAD BIKES ARE EFFICIENT

Once you get the hang of a road bike you can ride it for a really long time. In fact, you'll have no problem taking off on it for the better part of a day. To all outward appearances, you're not doing much besides pumping the pedals, but as you ride, your body is interacting with the bicycle to an extraordinarily nuanced degree. You're in tune with the road surface and unweighting ever so slightly to account for irregularities in the pavement. You're shifting your body fore and aft on climbs and descents. You're leaning into turns, countersteering and generally engaging in all sorts of complex physics without even thinking about it, for hours at a time.

At the same time, because your rides are getting longer and longer, you're building your strength and endurance. You're also learning about your body—how and when to feed and water it, how it functions on different types of fuel, and how to recognize the first signs of exhaustion and breakdown.

These are the things that make you good at riding a bike. And yes, you're doing this stuff on any type of bicycle, but on a more comfort-oriented bike you're not so much becoming one with the road as you are sopping it up like it's tomato sauce and the bike is a big hunk of semolina bread.

Other Types of Drop-Bar Bikes
CYCLOCROSS BIKES

The sport of cyclocross has become increasingly popular and so have the bikes. Cyclocross bikes are basically road bikes that have been optimized for riding through grass, dirt, sand, and mud, and this makes them particularly versatile.

It can be difficult for the novice to tell a cyclocross bike from a road bike because both have drop bars and share many common components, so here's a quick guide.

If the bicycle has knobby tires and cantilever or disc brakes, it's probably a cyclocross bike.

If the bicycle has slick tires, sidepull caliper brakes, and an extremely uptight rider on top, it's probably a road bike.

Caution: The recent advent of disc brakes on road bikes makes visual diagnosis more difficult, so to be absolutely sure simply rub dirt on the bicycle. If the owner freaks out, it's a road bike, and if the owner doesn't notice (or if the bicycle is already soiled), it's probably a cyclocross bike.

At this point you're probably wondering, "I'm a filthy slob. So does this mean I should get a cyclocross bike?"

Well, it depends.

While you can't go too wrong with a cyclocross bike, you may not need one either. The extra tire clearance and ability to ride more rugged terrain are good features, but the geometry and gearing may be less than ideal for the road, so if you'll be spending most of your time on pavement, then you should probably opt for a road bike. Also, note that true cyclocross racing bikes forgo extras like fender eyelets and occasionally even water bottle mounts, and this can cancel out a lot of the versatility you'd get from a road bike. Lastly, road bike brakes are generally a bit easier to adjust.

But if you think you'll be spending most of your time in the dirt yet you still want a fast bike, go ahead and try a cyclocross bike.

STUFF TO KEEP IN MIND WHEN SHOPPING

• FIT

The frame should fit you as well as possible. It's possible to compensate for a centimeter or two here or there, but you're going to get the most use and pleasure out of a well-fitting bike.

• TIRE CLEARANCE

Some road bikes have more tire clearance than others. If you can find a bike that has room for 28mm or even 32mm tires, then a simple tire swap can open up a whole new world of terrain to you. If there are clearance and eyelets for a set of real fenders, that's even better. Staying dry can make the difference between riding through the winter and succumbing to seasonal affective disorder. Remember: You don't *need* to use fat tires or fenders if you don't want to, but you might as well have the option.

• GOOD CLOTHES ARE WORTH MORE THAN GOOD COMPONENTS

When you're looking for a road bike you're bound to get hung up on all sorts of mind-numbing questions, like "Are the Super Attack shifters good enough or do I need to upgrade to the Super Attack Plus?" Forget it, it's not important. Your clothes, however, are hugely important. Remember, you're going to be spending hours at a time in a variety of weather

conditions on this contraption. Your fingers aren't going to care how many grams your shifter weighs, but you better believe your crotch will care what's between it and the saddle.

STUFF YOU DON'T NEED TO WORRY ABOUT

• ELECTRONIC SHIFTING

Save your money. You don't need it. Don't you have enough things to plug in and charge already?

• DISC BRAKES

I'm not saying there's anything wrong with disc brakes on road bikes; I'm just saying you don't need them. There are few components that are easier to adjust and maintain than rim brakes. Plus, when you consider that your wheel is essentially a great big rotor, you realize that rim brakes are disc brakes anyway.

• A REALLY LIGHT BIKE

Can you lift the bike easily off the ground? There you go. The bike is light enough.

TOURING BIKES

Does the countryside call out to you so loudly that you not only want to ride through it but also sleep in it? Are you perfectly comfortable using strange bathrooms, or even holes when proper facilities are not available? Do you scoff at the notion that cyclocross riders are "dirty" when you regularly forgo baths for several days? If you've answered yes to most of these questions, then the Wagon Queen Family Truckster of drop-bar bikes, otherwise known as a touring bike, is something to consider.

Touring bikes vary in wheel size and other specifications, and indeed they don't need to have drop bars at all—although they often do, as drop bars afford the multiple options for hand positions you'll want during hours upon hours in the saddle. They also have lots of eyelets for the racks and panniers you'll need to carry all your gear for day after day on the road.

These same features also make touring bikes potentially practical bikes for daily around-town use, and certainly there's no law that says that every time you hop on a touring bike you need to wind up in a tent beneath the stars. They're also inherently stable, which they need to be in order to carry all that stuff.

So if speed and maneuverability are less attractive to you than the prospect of escape, and if you regularly wear Birkenstocks, a touring bike may be for you.

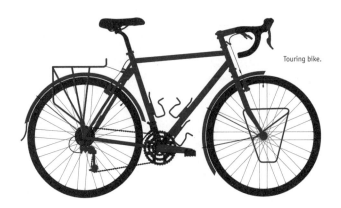

Touring bike.

MISCELLANEOUS "ADVENTURE" BIKES

It's hard to imagine a long-distance cycling situation in which you wouldn't be covered by a road bike, a cyclocross bike, or a touring bike.

Nevertheless, bike companies are constantly adding new types of drop-bar bicycles for increasingly specific uses. To wit, the growing popularity of the "gravel bike," which is essentially somewhere between a road bike and a cyclocross bike, two types of bicycles between which there wasn't much daylight to begin with.

Conversely, they're also coming up with drop-bar concepts for *less* specific uses. These bikes are usually called something along the lines of "adventure bikes," and they purport to be road bikes you can go touring on but also use in a cyclocross race because why the hell not?

While there's certainly no reason to avoid any of these bikes if they're appealing to you and well-suited to your lifestyle, it's also important to understand they can sometimes be branding exercises that are based on the long-running and well-established types of drop-bar bicycles above. Just make sure you're getting the features you want and not just some clever decals and an irreverent model name.

TRACK BIKES

Track bikes are specifically for velodrome racing, hence their single-gear ratio, lack of brakes, and inability to coast. This makes them about as ill-suited for road use as it's possible for a bike to be, because if there are three things it's handy to be able to do when riding on the road, they are stopping, shifting, and coasting.

Despite this—or, more likely, *because* of this—sometime around the early aughts track bikes became hugely popular among people who had recently arrived in the city from the suburbs, exurbs, or private colleges and wanted to look like bike messengers.

In the last several years, the track bike trend has largely subsided. Sure, there are die-hard hipsters still riding around the city

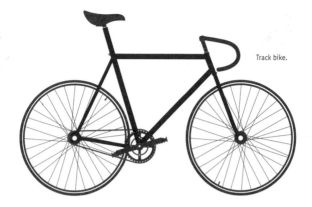

Track bike.

on track bikes, but as for the rest of the street trackies, they soon realized that "Hey, riding bikes is fun! You know what would make it even more fun? Having brakes and gears!" Then they bought cyclocross bikes.

So unless you actually want to race on a velodrome, skip the track bike—even if someone who has since learned better wants to sell it to you for cheap—because it's the cycling equivalent of wearing stilettos in a snowstorm.

MOUNTAIN BIKES

Look out your window and survey the landscape. What do you see? Mountains? Plains? Tundra? Whatever your local landscape, at some point you may be compelled to leave the road and venture out into it. If so, you'll want something called a mountain bike.

The term "mountain bike" is misleading, because only occasionally does off-road cycling involve riding on actual mountains. Mostly you're just on trails, though "trail riding" sounds far too relaxing and doesn't make for good marketing campaigns. Also, there's such a huge variety of mountain bike styles that it's almost silly to place them all under a single category. Road bikes are very simple in comparison because a road is, more or less, a road. But once you leave the road, it's a different story, for Mother Nature (or the Omniscient Celestial Bob Ross, as I prefer to personify nature) has painted us an infinite variety of landscapes, all of which call for different tire treads, geometries, suspension configurations, and so on.

Furthermore, nature's bounty has furnished the bike industry with a limitless canvas onto which it can endlessly paint innovations—some of which greatly improve the off-road riding experience, others of which are overpriced pieces of garbage, and the majority of which lie someplace in between.

Most of all, mountain biking is *hard*. Not hard in the sense that road biking is hard, but hard in the sense that it can sometimes be very difficult to even stay on the bike. Therefore, mountain bikers are often willing to pay for anything that promises to make riding even slightly easier and that will elicit admiring comments from other riders like, "Wow, how did you clear that?"

All of this is why, more than any type of bicycle, you should first attempt to purchase a *used* mountain bike. Fortunately you can do so very inexpensively, and here's why.

Various grizzled folk in California and Colorado have laid claim to the invention of the mountain bike. Some have gone on to reap untold wealth, while others have simply gone on to smoke untold amounts of weed. Regardless, what matters is that by the 1990s, the mountain bike had become the default variety of consumer bicycle. This is because mountain bikes have a rugged appearance, and Americans love stuff with wheels that look rugged.

Of course, while Americans may love rugged stuff, they almost never use it to *do* rugged stuff. This is why most Jeeps get no farther than the shopping mall parking lot, and most TAG Heuer watches go no deeper than the murky bottom of the resort hot tub.

Similarly, back in the 1990s, many Americans bought mountain bikes due to their robust appearance and promise of adventure, but relatively few of them heeded that call by seeking out trails. They also found that bikes with big knobby tires and flat handlebars are a literal and, therefore, figurative drag to ride on pavement, which is the terrain by which most of us are surrounded.

The upshot of all of this is that pretty much every garage and bike room in North America has at least one unused mountain bike in it—and if you ask nicely, you can probably get it for free. If the person you ask nicely can't find it, tell them to look behind the Jeep.

The other characteristic of the mountain bike that works in your favor is that the componentry becomes obsolete very quickly. For example, 26-inch wheels were the mountain bike standard for decades. Then 27.5- and 29-inch wheels came along, and suddenly now mountain bikers regard 26-inch wheels as tiny, useless, and diminutive. However, they're far from useless (as long as a wheel is round it is not useless), which means you can pick up an old 26-inch mountain bike for a song. (Though we are talking mountain bikes here, so it's probably a really bad song by some scuzzy bro-metal band.)

Suspension is another mountain bike component that's constantly evolving, which means you can get a bike equipped with older suspension technology very cheaply. Or better yet (because you never know when that old shock fork is liable to explode in a hail of shrapnel and oil), you can even pick up a bike with no suspension at all, often for next to nothing. Contrary to what most bike companies and many mountain bikers will tell you, it is indeed possible to ride off-road without shocks or suspension. In fact, depending on where you live it could be *easier*. You'd be surprised how many mountain bikers are wasting huge amounts of energy bouncing around on suspension they don't need. Most of all, riding without suspension makes you a better rider, which means you'll know exactly what you need when it comes time to buy a brand-new bicycle.

Here, generally speaking, are the main types of mountain bikes and what they're for.

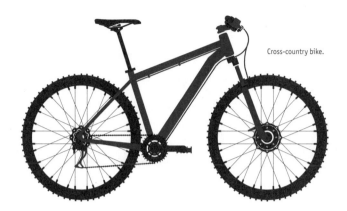

Cross-country bike.

CROSS-COUNTRY (OR "XC") BIKES

These bikes are for racing, or at least riding fast, on "cross-country" courses. So what does cross-country mean? Well, generally speaking, it means you might have to hop some logs or ride over some rocks, but you're not going to have to "catch air" or ride off drops that are taller than you.

If you prefer a spirited ride during which one or both of your tires maintain contact with the ground, then this is the mountain bike for you.

Cross-country bikes are lightweight and they generally have front suspension, though increasingly they have front and rear suspension—partially because technology has allowed bike companies to build dual-suspension bikes that are still light, but mostly because people are willing to pay for it.

TRAIL (OR "ALL-MOUNTAIN") BIKES

Okay, so you're not going to be launching yourself off of any cliffs, but you're also a bit more interested in jumping over and off of stuff than you are in scampering through the forest like a squirrel. You're also more inclined to wearing baggy shorts and jerseys, calling rides "sessions," and generally getting "stoked" about stuff with your bros or sisses.

To this end, a trail bike offers more suspension travel than a

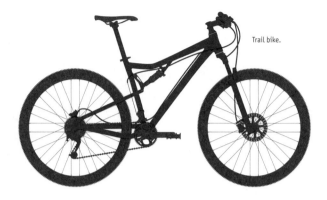

Trail bike.

cross-country bike (that means it moves more, thus soaking up bigger obstacles), and it also has a geometry more conducive to stability than to quick handling.

FREERIDE BIKES

The saddle height on a freeride bike is lower, the suspension is more absorptive, and the geometry is more conducive to keeping the bike stable while you're riding downhill than it is to lending you agility while climbing—which you don't do anyway, because you're not stoked on effort that doesn't immediately result in high-speed radness, dude.

When you go riding (sorry, "sessioning") you don't travel too

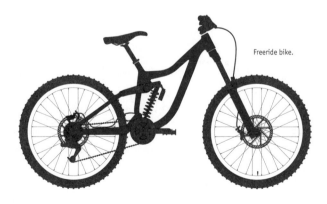

Freeride bike.

far, and instead linger around forbidding obstacles that you ride or jump off of over and over again (this is called "hucking," dude), perhaps while one of your bros or sisses shoots videos of you doing so. You're not terribly interested in going up hills, but you're, like, totally stoked on going down them, which is why you will ride a chairlift to the top of a mountain if it is available.

Your shorts and jersey are voluminous, and you probably wear shin and elbow protection too. You don't wear a lightweight vented racing helmet; instead you wear one of those solid ones that looks like a batting helmet. Generally speaking, you look like a hockey goalie.

DOWNHILL BIKES

Do you have a desire to tear down mountain slopes at terrifying speeds? Because a downhill bike needs to go in only one direction—and that's down—it has lots of suspension travel and looks like it has been stretched diagonally by pickup trucks driving in opposite directions.

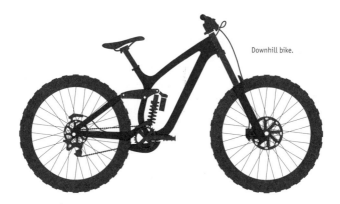

Downhill bike.

FAT BIKES

A few years ago people thought fat bikes were just a fad, but they're selling these things at discount chains now so it looks like they're here to stay.

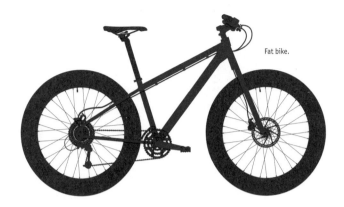

Fat bike.

A fat bike is simply a mountain bike with fat tires. *Really* fat tires, which can be ridden at extremely low pressures. Ostensibly, this allows fat bikes to float over terrain in which other mountain bikes would get mired, such as sand and especially snow.

For the time being, fat bikes are pretty simple mechanically, since the gigantic tires obviate the need for suspension. However, this is the bike industry we're talking about, so they're already available in exotic materials, and you can rest assured suspension is on the way.

Basically if you saw *Fargo* and thought it was a documentary, then you might want to consider a fat bike.

City Bikes

The general shape of road and mountain bikes is based not only on function but also on the rules put forth by the governing bodies of the sports in which they are used. You may never turn a pedal in competitive anger on your road or mountain bike, but chances are its general design is based on a racing bike of some kind and, therefore, is subject to the whims of the International Cycling Union (Union Cycliste Internationale, or UCI).

City bikes, on the other hand, are governed by little else than what works in a particular city. They are unique to their riders and tempered by various style guidelines and rules of thumb that come in and out of fashion as the years go by. In fact, there really is no such thing as a "city bike," besides the fact that lots of people ride bikes to get around cities—so if you're riding a bike in the city, then it is *ipso facto* a city bike.

Nevertheless, if you want to ride around your city or town and don't know where to begin, here are some of the city bikes you're most likely to come across and/or cobble together on your own.

STRIPPED DOWN

City bikes live a hard life. Locked to poles, pilfered, neglected, they're alumni of the School of Hard Knocks, and the stripped-down city bike is the valedictorian with a BA in Not Giving a Damn. Its tone is clipped; its physique is lean. Fenders? Yeah, right. Gears? Please, who needs 'em. Paint? Maybe three owners ago, but between the stickers and the scratches the color is now inde-terminate. At most, the stripped-down bike might have a pair of grips for comfort (be sure to say "comfort" condescendingly and

A note on wheel sizes

As I mentioned, larger wheels have mostly taken over on mountain bikes, and with good reason: The larger a wheel, the more capable it is of rolling over bumpy stuff, which is what mountain bikes are made to do.

If you're shopping for a new mountain bike, depending on the style, you will most likely be deciding between 27.5- and 29-inch wheels. So which is better? Well, the short answer is "Yes." I have my preferences, but I also don't live where you do. Your height is also a factor. This is why it's good to have a relationship with a bike shop.

As for those sad, diminutive, all-but-forgotten 26-inch wheels, you should absolutely not hesitate to buy a used bicycle equipped with them, provided it is cheap. We made 26-inch bikes work for years, and you can too. The worst thing that will happen is that in a few years you'll get a bike with bigger wheels and you'll totally be "stoked" about how easily it rolls over stuff.

Lastly, many fat bikes technically have 26-inch wheels, but the tires are so damn fat they don't count as 26ers.

then spit afterward), but just as likely the rider is now simply holding on to bare metal.

Bikes like this are generally made and not bought, in that they've been ridden for years and now all that's left are the barest essentials—but if you want to make one, here's how to do it:

1. Get a bike. Any bike.

2. Ride it a lot.

3. If a part breaks, falls off, or gets stolen and the bike becomes unrideable, replace that part as inexpensively as possible.

4. If a part breaks, falls off, or gets stolen but you can still ride the bike, just say, "Screw it" and keep going.

5. Before you know it you'll have a real stripped-down city bike . . . because it's been stripped down by *life*.

Still, plenty of companies will happily sell you a bare-bones street bike right off the rack. So if you like the idea of prosaic and utterly defrilled urban transport, but you don't have the time and patience to ride a bike into the ground in pursuit of authenticity, then you can certainly go the ready-made route. However, just know that a true urchin bike will see your store-bought model coming like "Ratso" Rizzo did Joe Buck.

GENTEEL

Okay, so the stripped-down bike isn't for you. You want a bike that's nice to look at. You want some extras. When you go to the farmer's market you want to be able to throw your canvas shopping bag into a basket. You want some fenders to keep dirt off your clothes, and maybe even something to cover the drivetrain so you don't have to worry about your leg getting greasy.

Nothing wrong with a little dignity.

Fortunately, as cycling for transportation becomes more popular, so do nicely designed yet inexpensive and practical bicycles. These will generally have features like fenders and chain guards, as well as tasteful aesthetics that will ensure the bike looks good when parked inside your open-plan office. They may or may not have multiple gears, which you may or may not need depending on where you live. They'll also have swept-back bars for comfort, yet still offer a degree of sporty maneuverability for weaving your way through all that gentrification.

If you've ever said, "I don't know what kind of bike I want. I just want a bike," then this is probably the bicycle for you.

SPORTING

Way back in the late twentieth century the bicycle industry came up with something called the "hybrid bike," which was basically a cross between a road bike and a mountain bike. Hybrids had the large wheels, light weight, and taller gearing of a road bike, yet they had the flat bars, wider tires, and the increased frame clearance of a mountain bike. These bikes were aimed squarely at the suburbanite who wanted something to ride on the bike path while wearing noncycling-specific workout gear, and in a way they're the quintessentially American bicycle.

Today, most companies have abandoned the term "hybrid." However, the *idea* of the hybrid—a sporty, go-anywhere bike that is neither full-on roadie or all-terrain bike—is still going strong, and most bike companies offer one under some contrived-sounding category like "x-road" or "path" or "multi-use."

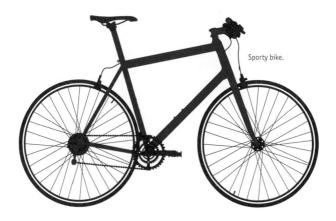

Sporty bike.

The reason the hybrid not only still exists but also remains very popular (albeit under various rebranded guises) is because the idea is sound: They're comfortable, they're versatile, and they can do pretty much anything, provided it isn't racing or super-aggressive riding. Throw on some workout clothes and you're ready for that charity ride; fit a rack and some fenders and you've got a solid commuter. Or strip it down and you've got a pretty lean city bike.

Of course, today's hybrids have more modern features, such as disc brakes and shaped frame tubing, but thanks to their *fin de siècle* ubiquity you can probably pick up a used one at a yard sale for about what a new helmet costs these days.

DUTCH

The trickiest thing about choosing a bicycle is not knowing exactly how you're going to wind up using it. Maybe you like the idea of cycling, but you don't know if you're going to end up doing it for fitness or adventure or commuting or maybe even all three. Therefore, you're likely to opt for something sporty and versatile.

If, however, you know precisely what you want out of a bike, and that's getting around your relatively flat city at a comfortable

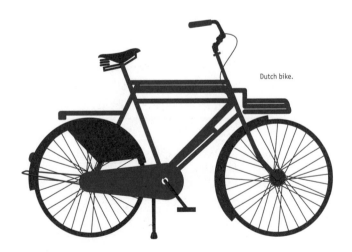

Dutch bike.

speed without making any kind of a fuss about it, then what you want is a Dutch bike—or, as the Dutch call it, a bike.

Netherlands is sort of a strange parallel universe where people embrace something called "common sense" when it comes to transportation, and so they use bicycles to travel short distances. These bikes are simple, comfortable, and robust. Quite often they are black. They have racks for carrying both inanimate objects and human children. (Yes, you can carry a human child on a rack, just like groceries.) They also have chain guards and skirt guards, and internal gearing to keep your clothing from getting stuck—that's your regular, everyday clothing, because common sense dictates that you don't need special clothing just to pedal a bike for a couple of miles at a time.

If you're dressed appropriately for the weather, that doesn't change just because you hop onto something with wheels. Also, changing your clothes at the office negates all the time you saved by riding a bike in the first place, doesn't it?

Another thing you don't do when riding a Dutch bike is bring it inside your home afterward. Keeping a Dutch bike inside is like a farmer keeping a milking cow in the living room instead of in the barn. Also, Dutch bikes are heavy, because when it comes to bikes, there's an inverse relationship between "light" and "practical." What good is saving a few grams if your pants get caught in your chain because of it? Therefore, should you attempt to carry your Dutch bike up the stairs in the evening after having a few drinks with friends, your neighbor might find you the next day trapped underneath it, your lifeless fingers just a few inches shy of your smartphone.

Unfortunately, the Dutch bike isn't a viable choice in certain parts of the world, such as much of North America. This is partly an issue of geography (hills and Dutch bikes don't go well together), but mostly because we've worked very hard over the years to design any sort of accessibility out of our cities and roadways and to cram as many cars into them as possible. Therefore, the fussless inertia of a Dutch bike may not work where you live, because Dutch bikes work best when you have amenities like bike lanes and racks for parking.

Sadly, when it comes to transportation, sporting bikes still have the edge in many places simply because they make it a bit easier to quickly maneuver your way out of a jam.

The other issue with Dutch bikes is that they're not always readily available in North America, and because they're not all that common here, they've become something of a luxury item.

If, however, you have the convenience of both flatness and bike infrastructure in your city or town, the Dutch bike could be the purposeful bike of your practical dreams.

CARGO BIKES

If you want to carry a few things, it's fairly simple to equip most types of bicycles with accessories like baskets or racks or kiddie seats.

If, however, you want to carry the kid and the kid's bike and three bags of groceries, *and* you want to stop at the wine store too—all without worrying about where you're going to put everything—what you need is a cargo bike.

Cargo bikes can be life-changing, because they allow you to dispense with the planning that riding a bicycle for transportation and errand running can sometimes require. Now, you can just buy

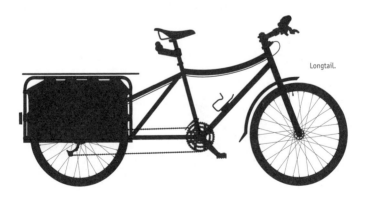

Longtail.

whatever and throw it right in the bike, just like you would with a car. This is good because it's convenient, but if you're not careful it can also be bad, because now your car isn't the only place you're liable to find a six-month-old half-eaten box of doughnuts.

There are lots of different kinds of cargo bikes, but here are two of the most common:

1. LONGTAILS. These look like regular bikes that have been stretched, and they usually feature some combination of platforms and bags for cargo behind the rider. The advantage of longtails is that they ride more or less like regular bikes, which can be an advantage in less bike-friendly cities where you don't want to dispense with maneuverability. They're also fairly well suited to longish rides. The disadvantage is that carrying large loads can require a bit of creativity. Also, it's harder to keep an eye on what you're carrying or to carry on a conversation with an inquisitive child passenger when the load is behind you.

2. BAKFIETS. These are basically great big tubs on wheels. Storing human and nonhuman cargo alike is as easy as just throwing it in the tub—a child can even curl up in one and go to sleep. The advantages here are simplicity and stability. The disadvantages are extra width and more deliberate handling. If you live in a crowded city without bike lanes you will have a tough time threading a

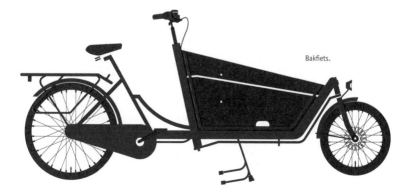

Bakfiets.

bakfiets through traffic. Also, if there are any hills around you and the bakfiets is not fitted with some sort of motor assist, you will soon want to kill yourself, or at least lease a Hyundai.

FOLDING BIKES

Folding bikes make a lot of people uncomfortable—and not only because riding a bike with tiny wheels makes you look a little like a circus bear.

No, folding bikes make people uncomfortable because they obviate pretty much every excuse people make for not using bikes as transportation.

"I'd ride a bike, but I have nowhere to park it."

"I'd ride a bike, but I don't want it to get stolen."

"I'd ride a bike, but I don't want to get stuck in the rain."

And so forth.

With a folding bike, you don't have to worry about any of that stuff. No room at home? A folding bike fits in a closet. Worried about bike theft? Tuck it under your desk. Not interested in braving foul weather? When the storm clouds start gathering just fold the thing up and hop on a bus.

You can even throw your folding bike into the trunk of your car if you want, because there's no rule that says you can't combine cycling with driving.

In fact, despite their disparate sizes, folding bikes and cargo bikes are very similar in that they both take a lot of the thought and planning out of riding a bicycle. You don't really have to worry about carrying tools or spare inner tubes or water bottles or a raincoat when you ride a folding bike, because if anything goes wrong all you really have to do is fold it up and become a pedestrian again.

And while folding bikes do handle a bit differently than "normal" bikes, they're still quite capable and can do pretty much anything "normal" bikes can. And what they may lack in handling, they make up for with the fact that you can bring them pretty much anywhere.

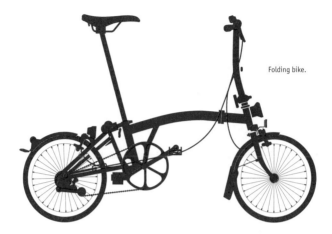

Folding bike.

Indeed, when you press people on why they object to folding bikes, it almost always comes down to matters of aesthetics. Sure, some are "cooler" than others, but yes, if you admire and covet the sleek design of full-size bicycles, then a folding bike—what with its unsightly hinges and accessory-like personality—can have all the appeal of a set of nail clippers.

But once you actually use a folding bike for a while, you come to appreciate its utility, and the fact that all that dorkiness can fold and unfold itself into something resembling elegance.

Recumbents and Other Rethinkings of the Bicycle

So far, all of the bikes I've described are based on the same principle: two in-line wheels and an upright rider. There's a reason for this, which is that this design *works*. In fact, apart from the bakfiets and the folders, pretty much all of these bikes have a diamond frame and two same-size wheels in common, and the differences between the various bike styles mostly come down to geometry and accessories.

Still, there are those for whom the tried and true is not appealing. They tried it, and they deemed it false. We all know people like this. They prefer the new *Star Wars* movies to the old ones.

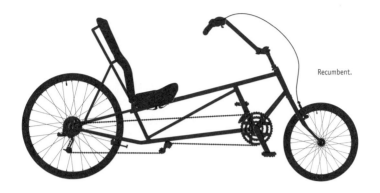

Recumbent.

They keep ferrets instead of cats. They're willing and eager to wear Google Glass in public.

For these people, there exist . . . alternatives.

The best-known alternative bicycle design is the recumbent—that's the one that looks like a bobsled on wheels. Why ride such a bike?

Recumbent bicycles do have their advantages. They dispense with the upright seating position that causes some riders much crotch discomfort. They're very efficient, which is why they're used in pursuit of the human-powered land speed record. You're also highly unlikely to go over the bars and land on your head while riding one, for the same reason you're probably not going to fall on your face while you're lying in bed.

And, of course, for those with disabilities, a three-wheeled recumbent can be the difference between riding and not riding.

E-BIKES

We're now officially living in The Future, which means pretty much all the bicycles above can be outfitted with some sort of electrical assist.

Cyclists have strong feelings about putting motors of any kind on bikes, because not only is human power one of the defining characteristics of the bicycle, but it's also the source of almost all rider smugness. This is why cyclists get annoying piston tattoos on their calves and brag about the size of their freakish quads. Therefore, to many cyclists, a motorized bicycle is as inherently self-contradictory as a veggie burger with bacon.

Nevertheless, there's no denying we're living in a time of great technological advancement. So why shouldn't you let it help you along a bit?

There are all different kinds of e-bikes, and they range from "normal" bikes that offer a little help to great big landspeeders you barely have to pedal and that look like a personal mobility scooter crossed with a Vespa. (You may have dodged one of the latter on the sidewalk recently, as they're often used for delivering food.)

It's probably inevitable that e-bikes will become more and more popular, because if there's one thing true of humanity, it's that we're always looking for ways to expend less effort. In the meantime, while ethics require I urge you to partake of your velocipeding unassisted if at all possible, here is a list of scenarios in which you might consider an e-bike, from most to least justifiable:

• **Physical considerations.** E-bikes make it possible for people to ride who might not otherwise be able to, such as the elderly. If you've almost been hit by a '76 Buick with Florida plates and an invisible driver I'm sure you'd agree that a world in which the elderly have ready access to bicycles is preferable.

• **Food delivery professional.** If your livelihood depends on delivering food by bicycle, then certainly you should be entitled to augment that with a little mechanical help—as long as you stay the hell off the sidewalk.

• **Adverse environment.** So you want to get around by bike, only you live on the edge of a mountain or in a desert or some other kind of forbidding hellscape where gravity or heat or some combination thereof makes riding for transportation nearly impossible. If it's the difference between riding and not riding, then why not?

• **Giant cargo bike.** There are cargo bikes so big that sometimes the chief limiting factor is your ability to propel it up a tiny incline. If you're regularly carting three children, the family groceries, and a bullmastiff, then people should look the other way if you opt for a little mechanical tailwind—especially when most people are riding around in four-wheeled recumbents with two-hundred-horsepowered gasoline assists, satellite radio, and air-conditioning.

• **Recreational cycling.** This one's the least defensible—and maybe even indefensible—if you are an able-bodied human. I mean, come on; you're supposed to be doing this for fun! The least you could do is pedal the bike! Do you want someone to spoon feed your lunch to you after the ride too? If you want to ride a bike with a motor, then just take up motorcycling.

Probably the most alarming development has been the advent of the mountain e-bike. Ethical considerations aside, do unfit riders really need help getting higher up mountains or deeper into the woods? Lousy riders don't need their lousiness amplified. It's like giving a crappy guitar player a Stratocaster and a Marshall stack—at least with an acoustic you can shut the door and tune them out. You don't want an e-assist mountain bike for the same reason you don't want a surfboard with a motor on it—paddle out to catch a wave and before you know it you're marooned on an island somewhere.

STUFF

One of the more intimidating aspects of cycling is that you need a lot of stuff—or at least that's what your coworker who does triathlons is always telling you.

The truth is that you don't really need all that much stuff to ride a bike. In fact, thanks to bike share programs in many cities you don't even really need a bike anymore. (In New York City it's now five times easier to find a bike than a public restroom.) What you need and how much you need really depend on how you're using the bike, and a lot of this is subjective anyway, because while most people would agree that you should invest in a proper pair of cycling shorts if you're going to ride a century, I'm sure there are plenty of hardy, reptilian-crotched souls who are more than happy to tackle one hundred miles while going commando in a pair of jorts.

Anyway, Mr. or Ms. Leathercrotch notwithstanding, here are some basic items you really should purchase along with your bike. For simplicity's sake, I'm categorizing them under "fun riding," "practical riding," and "all riding."

Fun riding: This is riding simply for the sake of riding. Whether it's competing in the Masters National Road Championships or lighting out for a three-day bike tour, you're doing this for you and your own personal satisfaction.

Practical riding: Going to work. Going to school. Going shopping. Yes, even making a social engagement. The point is you're moving your life forward, however slightly, and once the ride is over you've accomplished something.

All riding: You put a bike under you and you pedal it somewhere.

By the way, it's important to remember that practical riding can (and should) also be fun, while so-called "fun riding" can totally suck, which is why roadies always scowl.

Fun Riding
TOTALLY NECESSARY

✔ HELMET. We'll have "the helmet talk" later. For now, let's just say that cycledom and our culture in general have probably invested more stock in bicycle helmets than is warranted.

Frankly, I don't care if you wear a helmet or not. Nevertheless, if you're going to be riding for recreational purposes—by which I mean wearing special clothes and cycling for hours at a time o'er hill and dale—you really should have one. If nothing else, you never know when you're going to cross into some park or munici-pality where there's a rule in place requiring you to wear one, and haggling with law enforcement is a poor use of your riding time.

Also, sooner or later you're going to want to take part in some sort of organized cycling event, and whether it's a charity ride or a race, pretty much all of them require participants to wear a plastic hat.

✔ **SHORTS AND JERSEY.** If you're new to cycling, you might be self-conscious about wearing stretchy bike clothes. I don't blame you. Putting on cycling clothing for the first time feels like bringing your college boyfriend or girlfriend home to meet your parents: You don't know whether to be proud or embarrassed, though the look on everybody's face usually says it all.

Nevertheless, whether you plan to ride on- or off-road, you should at least own a jersey as well as a proper pair of cycling shorts with a padded "chamois," which are to be worn without underwear. The jersey will keep you cool and comfortable by wicking sweat away, and you'll have three handy pockets in back so you can reach for a banana without stopping. As for the shorts, if you're grinding away on the bike for hours at a time, you don't want your cotton underwear grinding away at your inner thighs.

You don't *have* to wear them if you don't want to, and if you prefer to ride around in a T-shirt and jeans, then by all means go right ahead. In fact, a lot of the time that's all you need. Sooner or later, though, you'll be tempted to ride farther and longer, and when you do you'll be grateful for the Lycra in your drawer.

✔ **WATER BOTTLES.** When you're cycling, dehydration doesn't announce itself. What happens is that you're riding along enjoying the summer sunshine, and then you start seeing stars, and then it's too late.

Your brain is dried out.

If you're able to make it home, you'll spend the next twelve to twenty-four hours nursing what feels like a hangover, which is especially unfair since you didn't even get to enjoy being drunk first. If you don't make it home or get picked up by an ambulance, you'll eventually die, and buzzards will pick at your eyeballs and flesh.

Therefore, if you're going to be spending multiple hours at a time on your bike outside of a city or town, you need to have water with you at all times. So be sure you have a convenient way to carry it. At the very least, make sure you leave the shop with a couple of water bottles and cages.

If you're going mountain biking, you might consider opting for a hydration pack instead. Perhaps you've seen them and wondered why people use these things, since they look like those *Dune* suits that recycle your bodily fluids for drinking. Well, here are the advantages:

- Large fluid capacity
- Allows you to drink without taking your hands off the bars
- Keeping stuff in the backpack
- Nozzle stays clean because it's far from the mud and dirt that gets thrown up by your tires

The main disadvantage is maintenance—specifically that the bladders require frequent cleaning or else they get moldy and disgusting. (Handy tip: Store bladder in the freezer.)

Also, if you're wondering why people don't use hydration packs for road riding, it's partially because it's nice not to have any extra stuff on your body when you're climbing up hills, but it's mostly a fashion thing. Still, there's no reason not to do so if the idea appeals to you and if you find it comfortable.

TAKE IT OR LEAVE IT

CLIPLESS PEDALS. If you've been thinking about taking up cycling for sport, you've almost certainly had somebody talk your ear off about the importance of foot retention, and about how all "serious" cyclists use clipless pedals.

Next time this happens, tell them to shut up.

What are clipless pedals? They're special pedals that attach to your special shoes. Basically your shoe has a cleat on its sole, and your pedal has springs that allow it to grip that cleat, and when you step on the pedal in just the right way the pedal grabs the cleat. We call this "clipping in."

If you've ever gone skiing you're familiar with the concept.

Why are they "clipless" if you "clip in" to them? Because before they were clipless, racing pedals had metal baskets screwed onto them, called "toe clips." You stuck your foot into the metal basket and then lashed it to the pedal with a leather strap. Imagine muzzling a dog and you've got the idea.

The reason behind clipless pedals (and the toe clips that preceded them) is that when your feet are stuck to your pedals, you're transferring as much energy as possible from your legs to the bicycle's transmission during every part of the pedal stroke.

It is true that most "serious" cyclists (or at least the ones who take themselves seriously) use clipless pedals, and it's also true that they can be quite helpful when it comes to riding quickly. Moreover, when you're riding a mountain bike, it can be much easier to hop the bike over obstacles when your feet are connected to the pedals.

As time goes on you will probably want to get yourself some clipless pedals.

But, really, you don't need to care. The simple fact is that bikes work just fine when you pedal them in your sneakers. Furthermore, it can take a while to get the hang of clipless pedals, and you are guaranteed to fall over with your feet still attached at least once or twice while you're learning how to use them. Given all the other stuff you'll be learning as a new cyclist, there's absolutely no reason to bother with clipless pedals until you feel like it—assuming you ever feel like it.

Much more important, don't let any of these foot-retention doofuses talk you into using toe clips, which still exist. The only way toe clips offer you any foot retention is if you wear special shoes with notched soles and lash your foot to the pedal so tightly that you have to bend down and release the strap in order to remove your foot again. Otherwise, all you're doing is wiggling your foot in and out of a stupid shoe muzzle completely unnecessarily. It's basically like wearing decorative suspenders. The awkwardness of toe clips is why they invented clipless pedals in the first place. It's like skipping the safety bicycle and going back to the penny farthing.

Practical Riding
TOTALLY NECESSARY

✔ **A LOCK.** If there's even the slightest chance you'll be parking your bike on the street, the second-most important thing after learning to ride your bike is learning how to lock it. I'll tell you how in detail later on in this book.

For now, let's just say *get a lock right away*—and not just any lock, either. Ask someone at the bike shop (that's *bike shop*, not bike department of your local big-box department store) for the best lock they sell, and then buy it. Don't even look at the price, just pay whatever it costs.

Again, buy the lock from a *bike shop*. Even if you bought your bike mail order or secondhand or three aisles over from the gardening supplies. Why? Because every day your local shop hears tales of woe from bike theft victims, and they've got a sense of what works in your area and what doesn't.

Even a tip offered in passing by a kid in a bike shop can be the difference between keeping your bike and losing it.

✔ **ANOTHER LOCK.** But wait, you're not done! Now you need *another* lock. Don't worry, this one doesn't have to be too expensive. In fact, ideally this second lock will be a cable lock, and those are generally pretty cheap. This auxiliary lock will serve two purposes:

1. It lets you secure stealable items, such as wheels or your saddle, in addition to the frame.

2. It requires more work on the part of the thief, which makes it that much less likely that the thief will go for your bike, because

when you're committing a crime, every second counts.

Using two locks may sound like a pain, but it's still a lot more convenient than walking outside and finding your bike gone.

✔ **LUGGAGE.** Obviously if you're going to work or school, or if you're running errands, then you're going to need to carry stuff from time to time. There are two ways to do this: with your body or with the bike.

With your body:
The noncycling world calls this technique "carrying a bag."
No fancy artisanal handmade-in-a-Mission-District-basement messenger bag necessary; pretty much any backpack will do.
—*Advantage:* Simple, cheap, less time loading and unloading bike, just hop on or off and go
—*Disadvantage:* Possible discomfort, limit to how much you can carry safely, big sweat stain on your back

With your bike:
Saddlebags, panniers, handlebar bags, baskets, and racks all allow you to load up the bike instead of yourself
—*Advantage:* Leaves your torso unencumbered and free, more load-carrying capacity, you show up at work with a clean shirt
—*Disadvantage:* Futzing around at the bike rack, bike tipping over while you're loading it, requires racks and attachments that may be difficult or impossible to fit to your bike depending on what you're riding

Of course, if you think you'll be carrying stuff regularly, you should make sure to buy a bike that allows you to fit racks and bags to it; if it's too late and you've got some sort of racy bike with limited braze-on and clearance, then you may be limited to the bag.

Whichever you choose, if you're commuting regularly it's

also a good idea to fit some kind of simple rear rack, which even a road or track bike will generally accept, though you might need some p-clamps if your frame doesn't have any eyelets preinstalled, or else one that bolts onto your seat post. This way there's always someplace to strap that unwieldy item that unexpectedly comes into your possession, like the leftovers from dinner.

✔ **STRAPS OR BUNGEE CORDS.** For the rack, of course! Always keep one or two in your bag or wrapped around your rack. You'll be thankful for them when you decide to swing by the wine store on the way home, and so will your dinner partner.

✔ **A JACKET.** If you were brought up right, then whenever you leave the house you should always hear a nagging voice in your head asking, "Did you bring a jacket?"

"But it's like ninety degrees!" you shout to nobody, eliciting stares from passersby.

Doesn't matter. Bring something—a Windbreaker, a sweater, a sweatshirt, anything. What if it rains? What if you stay out later than you expected? What if a bird craps all over your shirt when you're on your way to a social engagement and you need something to salvage your dignity?

Plus, a jacket has all kinds of additional uses, like sitting on in the park or padding the bottle of wine you're about to strap to your bare metal rack. You can even use it to *tie* stuff to your rack with the sleeves.

You're a cyclist; be resourceful!

✔ **A BELL.** I know what you're thinking: "I'm going to be 'sharing' the road with two-ton sound-insulated vehicles with blaring horns and roaring motors. What good is a dainty, diminutive bell?"

Well, for one thing, in many places you're required by law to have a bell on your bike, and if nothing else, you don't want to give the police any excuses to ticket you.

For another, yes, you're right—the typical motorist can't hear a bell over the stereo or the scraping of their own nose picking. However, where the bell is useful is in communicating with pedestrians.

Consider, for example, the shared path. Let's say you want to pass a group of pedestrians walking three abreast. Well, you could shout, "On your left!" thus consigning yourself to the ranks of all the other impatient doofuses zigzagging through crowded spaces and otherwise annoying people. Or you could emit a delightful Zen-like chime from the bell on your handlebars, thereby simultaneously gaining the pedestrians' attention and totally blissing them out. Then, as you pass, you give a friendly wave, and—hey, look at that—you've made a friend!

All Riding
TOTALLY NECESSARY

✔ **LIGHTS.** Drivers aren't attentive enough to avoid running into each other let alone cyclists. You are invisible to them until you're under their bumper, at which point they tell the police you "came out of nowhere," which probably comes as a surprise to you as you were at work all day and not in a state of Schroedinger-esque quasi-nonexistence in some alternate reality.

And that's just during the day. At night, without lights on your bike, even drivers *looking* for you (and, let's face it, like quarks, such drivers only exist in theory) have a hard time seeing you.

Therefore, lights are the most important thing you can put on your bike—besides tires (obviously) and a saddle (ouch). Moreover, you need the *right* lights—specifically a white one in the front and a red one in the rear, just like on cars.

Lots of people say screw it and put the red one on the front or vice versa, but when you do that, nobody can tell which way you're going, and the effect on drivers and other cyclists is psychedelic, disorienting, and, most of all, annoying, like watching a mime pretend to walk against the wind.

If you don't have lights permanently installed on your bike (which you may not want to do because people like to steal them) then you should always have at least one pair in your bag at all times, ready to fire up. This is much easier nowadays, since lots of companies sell USB-rechargeable lights, so all you need to do is plug them into your computer while you're pretending to work.

As a matter of etiquette, if you're using a particularly bright front light and you're riding someplace where there's lots of bike traffic, angle it down slightly—not enough so that drivers can't see it, but just enough so it's not shining directly into your fellow cyclists' eyes and searing their retinas.

✔ TOOLS. Unless you're not going beyond walking distance of your home, you should always carry a basic set of tools so that only the most serious mechanical failure will leave you stranded. We'll get into what the most likely breakdown scenarios are and how to fix them later, but for now, make sure you have the following:

• **Allen wrenches:** You can assemble and disassemble most bikes with little more than a set of Allen wrenches. The mini tool kits behind the register at your local bike shop include all the common sizes.

• **Tire repair supplies:** At least one (1) replacement tube *and* a set of patches, because if you flat more than once you should still be covered. Additionally, be sure to carry a set of tire levers in case you need help getting the tire off the rim. Perhaps most important, you need to be able to get air in there, so carry a pump. Not just a one-shot CO_2 inflator, but a *pump*, so that you can use it over and over and over again if necessary.

With a tiny box of six patches, two spare tubes, and a pump, you've got insurance against eight flats, which is more than you're likely to experience in a year.

Without any of this, you're calling someone to come pick you up.

• **Whatever you need to get your wheel on and off:** Study your bike. Does removing either the front or rear wheel require some additional tool not mentioned above, such as a fifteen-millimeter wrench? If so, make sure you have one at all times, because it's extremely difficult and annoying to repair a flat without removing your wheel.

CHOOSING A BIKE SHOP

We're a consumer culture. Buying stuff is more than just the basis of our economy. It's our religion. Our possessions define us. That's why we obsess over which logo is on the stuff we buy.

But when it comes to your cycling happiness, where you buy your bicycle is far more important than which one you buy. This is why you shouldn't worry so much about shopping for a bike. What you should focus on is shopping for a bike *shop*.

Having read the previous pages of this book, you now have a decent idea of what kind of bikes are available to you. Now you're probably wondering which *brand* is the best. Forget it. The truth is, real bike shops don't sell lousy bikes, and a good one knows how to put you on the one you need. Go shop shopping and let them guide you the rest of the way.

So how do you pick a bike shop? Well, just as you need to be comfortable on your bike, you need to be comfortable in the bike shop. Don't focus too much on their prices—feeling at home in the place you're buying your bike is more important. What good is saving $20 or $40 on a bike if you walk in stressed and walk out in a huff?

Until recently, bike shops were often intimidating places—a mélange of record store nerdiness and auto repair machismo. If you didn't know the right word for something, you were afraid to ask for it, and if you needed something fixed, you feared the bill—assuming they didn't look at your bike, declare it a piece of garbage, and laugh at you until you bought a new one.

This has changed considerably in the twenty-first century. Everything is kinder and gentler now. Dive bars are no longer dives;

they're *reclaimed*. Similarly, bike shops are often far more inviting than their twentieth-century counterparts. (And presumably the nineteenth-century ones too, where heaven forbid you were to walk in wearing an inferior blend of tweed.) When you bring your bike in for a repair it no longer disappears into a basement or back room; more often the mechanic works on it right there in an open area on the shop floor, and they even let you ask them questions and learn about what they're doing.

More important, there are now many different *styles* of bike shop to match all these different kinds of bikes. Here are some of the more common ones and how to identify them.

The Pro Shop

The first clue you're in a pro shop is obviously the bikes themselves—if you see lots and lots of carbon fiber, you're standing on the threshold of a stratospherically expensive realm of extreme perfectionism.

The next thing you're likely to notice are the multi-thousand-dollar wheelsets, and the wall of shoes, and the glass case full of baubles, gizmos, and componentry exotica.

Should you be compelled to press on, you'll also find certain luxury services available to you. Just as the high-end department store offers tailoring and spa service, the pro shop offers you premium services such as bike fittings—not the "stand over the bike"-type fittings you get at regular shops, but the "laser beams and computers"-type fittings done by technicians who are trained in proprietary techniques with names that have umlauts in them.

Then there are the coaches, who are usually affiliated with certain pro shops. Sure, you could ride your bike when you feel like it, but why do that when a coach will create a custom-tailored fitness-optimized schedule just for you? Coaches will tell you what to ride, when to ride, how to ride, and what to wear while you're doing it. They'll also work with the shop to fit both you and your bike with all manner of electronic devices so you can keep track of every pedal stroke.

Then they will send you an invoice.

In the world of the pro shop, the bike is sometimes the cheapest part.

The Bro Shop

It's a little bit like the pro shop—the stuff is expensive—but it's also a lot . . . cooler. Not "we're too busy to talk to you" cool, but "do I have enough tattoos to be in here?" cool. The bros in the bro shop are less about getting aero and more about getting "rad." There's more of an "indie" vibe than in the pro shop, and you'll find handmade bikes and boutique gear instead of imported carbon, but there's still a competitive undercurrent beneath it all.

The Corporate Shop

Some bike companies are bigger than others, and the biggest work with dealers that dispense their merchandise prominently, and sometimes almost exclusively. If you walk into a shop and everything from the bikes to the helmets to the socks to the gloves has the same brand name on it, then you're in a corporate shop.

I should stress that there is *nothing inherently wrong with a corporate shop*. Even the biggest bike company is not exactly Halliburton. We're talking *bicycles* here. How evil could a bike company possibly be?

Furthermore, if you're new to cycling, the advantages of a corporate shop are as follows:

- They have pretty much everything and they've got outfitting you down to a science.
- The service is generally friendly, because big companies don't want new customers receiving the *High Fidelity* treatment. Otherwise you say "forget bikes" and go shopping for a Hyundai.
- Shops that sell a lot of one company's stuff have good relation-

ships with that company, which means if you buy something and it breaks they'll probably be able to fix or replace it for you pretty quickly.

Sure, you may roll out looking like a cycling mannequin, but you're unlikely to go too far astray. It's like shopping at Banana Republic—nobody's going to mistake you for a rock star, but it's also pretty much impossible to look totally stupid.

The Hole in the Wall Where They Know Everything

At some point in your cycling life you are likely to encounter the archetypal bike sage who operates in a cluttered warren of a bike shop, dispensing wisdom, service, and arcane bike parts. Such shops have survived into the twenty-first century, and hopefully they'll continue to live on into the twenty-second and beyond. These shops are the opposite of the corporate shop. Sure, you might not find them in large numbers, and no, they may not be able to service your plutonium-powered twenty-second-century space bike, but they're your connection to cycling history, and in some cases they are museums unto themselves.

The Bike Boutique

Gentrification has brought the boutique shopping experience to bicycles, which means that the line between bike shop and haberdasher has become increasingly blurry. Now you can buy a bike or simply peruse neo-vintage leather accessories, woolen cycling garments, and off-the-bike clothing in the same establishment. If you'd rather be comfortable than fast, and you'd rather be stylish than anything, this is the place for you.

The Bike Café

Bikes and cafés have long gone together, and most rides start at one, finish at one, or visit one along the way. Traditionally, cafés and bike shops have been separate establishments, but increasingly proprietors have been fusing the two. Often the bike café is not a full-blown bike shop, but you can probably buy a tire or maybe even get a basic repair done while you're waiting for your cappuccino. There will also generally be lots of cycling memorabilia on display, usually in the form of jerseys and old racing bikes, and generally "curated" to make you feel like you're somewhere in Italy. The bike café is not a place to buy a bike so much as it is a place to point the bike once you've bought it.

The Bike Co-Op

If you're a member of a food co-op or a CSA you might want to think about joining your local bike co-op, where you can participate in workshops, access tool libraries, and volunteer your time to help your fellow cyclists.

If, however, you have your groceries delivered to your co-op apartment on Park Avenue, or you think a CSA is a type of financial instrument, you might be better off in the pro shop.

ESSENTIAL BIKE SHOP SURVIVAL SKILLS

Even in today's kinder, gentler retail landscape, people sometimes accuse bike shops of giving "attitude." Sometimes this may very well be the case, but just as often it's *you* who has the attitude.

Yeah, that's right, I'm looking at you.

Here are some things to keep in mind that will make your shopping experience as pleasant as possible.

Don't Be Insecure

Easier said than done, I know. "Have more self-confidence, dammit!!!" Sure, even the friendliest bike shop can be intimidating to the uninitiated. You're walking into a place filled with expensive stuff that you don't know anything about, and people you don't know are trying to sell it to you. So naturally you're defensive, and when the kid in the cycling cap tells you that you need to spend more money for the blah-blah-blah your first instinct is to protect your wallet and deflect this predatory salesperson with your kung fu moves.

Nevertheless, it's okay to let down your guard a bit and hear what they have to say. After all, it's a store. Believe it or not, usually they're actually trying to help you. Plus, their job is to sell you stuff; otherwise they don't eat. Look, *you* came to *them*! It's not like they're telemarketers bothering you at home while you're trying to binge watch on Netflix. And let's not lose sight of the fact that it's just a bike shop, not a hospital. What's the worst that's going to happen? We're talking about bikes, not unnecessary surgery.

None of this is to say you should buy everything they're selling, or indeed a*nything* they're selling. If you feel wrong about shelling out for something (or you plain don't have the money), then don't. At the same time, it's important to have an open mind and to let the bike shop present itself to you and offer you the kind of service it strives to provide.

It's like going on a first date with an oenophile—nobody's saying you have to marry them, but at least humor them by letting them order the wine.

The Customer Is *Not* Always Right

Not by a long shot.

How can you be right when you don't know anything?

Yes, the staff at a bike shop should always treat you with respect, but not if you insist you know something you don't.

Hey, not knowing anything is fine—as long as you're honest about it. It's when you pretend otherwise that you run into trouble. Here are ways to be wrong in a bike shop:

• **Insist that you're right about something because you "read it on the Internet."** People in bike shops interact with actual humans and touch stuff with their hands every day. So don't insult them by countering their well-meaning advice with something you read on a forum or on some dumb bike blog.

This goes double if you read it on your phone two seconds ago while standing in the store.

• **Demand free stuff.** Environmentalists have done us a disservice by convincing us that riding bicycles equals saving the Earth. Sure, bikes are clean and efficient, but the unintended side effect of this message is that you may now be under the impression that by purchasing a bicycle you are performing a public service.

You are not. For example:

Let's say you just bought a new bike. You've spent hundreds if not thousands of dollars on your clean, efficient form of green transportation. Shouldn't they at least throw in a free water bottle or a pair of socks?

No, they should not.

They spent half the day fitting you for that bike. The least you could do is buy some stuff to go with it.

• **Haggle.** And what about that bike you're buying? It has a tag with a number on it, right? Well guess what: *That's the price.*

If you like the shop and it's convenient, then why waste time arguing, and why run all over the place in search of a better deal? By all means, do your research and get a sense of what's a reasonable price, but don't drive yourself crazy over relatively small amounts of money.

Sure, you may save $20 at a shop that's farther away, but what happens when you need something fixed and you have to schlep all the way back just for a repair?

• **Request unnecessary service.** Generally, bike shops offer some sort of free tune-up during the "break-in period" of your bicycle. This can come in very handy. However, this does not mean you have to take them up on it if your bike is functioning properly. A bike isn't like a car, where you have to rigorously adhere to strict service schedules. In fact, even cars can go something like ten thousand miles between oil changes. So if your new bike is working fine, don't worry about it.

And if something isn't working right, take a few minutes to

try to address it yourself before asking the shop to do it for you. Really, this is less about sparing the bike shop the work than it is about educating yourself. Obviously you don't want to get in over your head, but sometimes that creaking or clicking is extremely simple to address, so take a look and see if you can figure it out. (You'll be a lot better equipped to do so after reading the "Understanding Your Bike" chapter of this manual.)

• **Expect fawning service when they're busy.** If your local bike shop is lucky, there are certain times when they are very busy, such as Saturday and Sunday afternoons in the spring and summer, or the day before the big charity ride.

Sometimes you need an inner tube and you need it now, in which case you may be forced to enter a busy bike shop during peak hours and elbow your way through the throngs of charity riders who wear their helmets indoors.

If, however, you're expecting someone to take the time to diagnose the faint ticking sound in your bottom bracket, you should come back another time.

When Buying a Bike, the Key Is Timing

If at all possible, visit the bike shop during the week. On Saturday afternoon the shop's staff is usually besieged by those charity riders. They're at the end of their wits.

However, by next Tuesday afternoon that same staff is bored and watching the same Paris-Roubaix DVD over and over again, so they will likely fall over themselves to help you. You'll have plenty of time to ask questions, have a conversation, and try out various bikes without losing your salesperson to another customer.

Better yet, buy your bike during the winter (assuming they have winter where you live). Winter is a great time to buy a bike because:

• The fair-weather cyclists are all in hibernation so the shop won't be crowded.

• The owner probably feels like Dave on the spaceship in *2001* and will likely be very happy to see you.

- You may land a great deal if the shop needs to clear the floor in anticipation of next season's new models—which are often the same as last season's models only with different decals.

"This All Seems Crazy to Me."

I know what you're thinking: "Why do I have to tiptoe around these people? These aren't my cranky in-laws; they're running a store! And I'm a paying customer!"

Very true. At the same time, a good shop is more than just a store—it's also something of a cultural hub. As your appreciation for cycling grows, your favorite shop may very well offer you guidance far beyond simply selling you stuff. Bike shops organize group rides. They sponsor racing teams. They support bike advocacy. The staff and customers of your favorite bike shop may very well become your closest friends, or at least your favorite riding partners.

BUYING USED

Okay, you're not buying your bike at a bike shop. There are no good shops around you, you don't have the money, etc.

It's true, lots of people buy bikes they never end up riding—or they buy new bikes and lose interest in the old ones—which in turn creates an opportunity for you to get lots more bike for your money.

At the same time, by venturing into the used-bike marketplace you are submitting yourself to a world that can be as sordid as it is irritating. If you've done your homework and you know your seller, then you may very well find that mythical top-of-the-line bike at an entry-level price. However, if you don't know what you're doing, you could find yourself getting extremely annoyed or just plain screwed.

First, here are the more common used-bike marketplaces, from most to least desirable.

Word of Mouth

This is the best way to buy a used bike. Your friend has "up-graded" and wants to sell you her old bike. Your coworker who does triathlons is selling his road bike because it's too practical for him. You're going to cut a little deal with your roommate.

You know what you're getting and everybody benefits.

Bike Community Classified List

Organizations such as bike clubs and owners' groups often buy and sell bicycles among themselves. This can be a good option because members of a community are generally more scrupulous in their dealings with one another—especially obsessive cyclists, who tend to be so neurotic that they feel compelled to disclose every flaw right down to the sticky chainlink they had to lube last week.

This is an especially good option if you covet a certain brand, because you can benefit from the passion of your fellow enthusiasts.

eBay

There isn't much you can't find on eBay. Plus, since you can view a seller's feedback, it's fairly unlikely you're going to get scammed (counterfeit goods notwithstanding), and pretty much impossible to get knifed.

However, the biggest danger with eBay is the addictive nature of auctions, something to which bike people in particular are highly susceptible thanks to our obsessive nature. What happens is that you find that bike you've been dreaming about, and there are no bids and no reserve. So you place your bid. In so doing, your brain releases a hit of endorphins, and you already feel like the bike is yours. You're glowing. You're riding it in your mind.

Then, days later, you get an e-mail. You've been outbid by some token amount. So you bid again. So do they. So do you. So does everyone else.

Why do they keep trying to take your bike?

So you bid and you bid and you bid again—the bike is yours after all—and before you know it you've got the bike, but you've paid too much for it, which defeats the purpose of buying a used bike in the first place.

Really, eBay is less a place for deals than it is a psychological kidnapper holding for ransom the bike stuff you covet.

Unless you've got a lot of restraint or you're looking for something incredibly specific, it's probably best to avoid it.

Craigslist

When it comes to trying to get stuff cheap, all roads eventually lead to Craigslist. Could your dream bike be waiting for you there at an unbelievable price? Sure it could. But to get it you'll have to brave the legions of the clueless and the delusional and the predatory and the deranged. Bikes on Craigslist generally fall under these categories:

- Bikes "customized" by people who are now selling them because they're unrideable.
- Recently purchased bikes for which the seller is asking pretty much what a bike shop would for a new one.
- Stolen.

In among all that is some genuinely good stuff, but it's fairly rare, since that stuff mostly gets sold to friends and fellow club members. (See Bike Community Classified List.)

If you're not already a bike expert, skip Craigslist.

The Guy on the Street Who Seems Really Anxious

Yeah, that bike's stolen. Legitimate businesspeople don't sell high-end bicycles for $50 because they "just really need a bus ticket." The only excuse for buying such a bicycle is if you're legitimately determined to reunite it with its owner. Otherwise, like anything in life that seems too good to be true, it involves drugs.

"WHY SHOULDN'T I BUY MY BIKE AT A DEPARTMENT STORE?"

There is no such thing as a bad bicycle. Sure, some are better than others, but the best bicycle is the one that gets ridden the most. Therefore, the department store bike you ride every day is a far better bicycle than the shiny custom one that gets ridden a few times during the season.

But be aware of a few things if you're purchasing a bike at a department store.

While Cheap, Not *That* Cheap

The $250 department store mountain bike may seem like a bargain compared to your local bike shop—until you consider there's no support network behind it. Sure, if there's something wrong with the bike they'll take it back, but that's where it ends. What happens a week after you buy the bike when you need some adjustments? (And you *will* need some adjustments, because department store bikes are not assembled to the same standard as bike shop bikes.) If you can't figure out how to adjust it yourself, then your only recourse will be to visit an actual bike shop, where they'll charge you for the labor since they didn't sell you the bike in the first place. In fact, once the bike shop mechanic corrects the store's assembly mistakes, you've probably spent almost as much as you would have if you'd bought a bike from the shop in the first place.

Inferior Quality

While there's no such thing as a bad bike, there is such a thing as a frustrating bike. The most expensive department store bike is often of lesser quality than the cheapest bike shop bike. I'm not talking about the more rarefied aspects of quality, such as weight or which alloy they used for the frame. I'm talking about basic stuff you'll notice right away, like inferior brakes that feel flexy and spongy, and wheels that don't stay true.

Bicycle marketing myths

• LIGHTER IS BETTER

You know what a light bike is good for? Carrying up the stairs. If you can do that without collapsing, then your bike is probably more than light enough.

It's pretty difficult to buy a genuinely heavy bike these days—unless the bike needs to be heavy by design, as is the case with cargo and Dutch bikes, in which case you're probably parking the thing outside anyway.

Gram counting and weight-weeniesm is a psychological disorder that can drain your wallet almost as quickly as a drug habit can. From a performance standpoint, the very best place to save weight is your midriff.

• FRAME MATERIAL DETERMINES RIDE QUALITY

A lot of people will try to tell you that you need a frame made out of a specific material in order to enjoy a comfortable ride. Usually this material is carbon fiber or titanium because—surprise!—they're the most expensive.

Of course, your frame material contributes to your bicycle's ride quality—that's *contributes*, not determines.

Tire width and air pressure are by far the most important factors in determining your bike's ride quality. Think about it: What's between you and the road surface? A cushion of air. The volume of that cushion is the first thing that informs the way your bike feels.

• BIKES ARE FAST

Wheel a bicycle out into the middle of your living room. Let it go and walk away. What happens?

It falls down—or, if it has a kickstand, it just stands there.

Either way, bikes are not fast.

Riders are fast.

Buy an appropriate bike for the style of riding you want to do. If you want to go faster, pedal accordingly. If you want to go still faster, keep working at it. The more you ride, the faster you get.

You can't buy speed. You can only buy the *appearance* of speed.

All of this means even an expert mechanic might not be able to get a department store bike to perform as well as a slightly more expensive bike shop bike.

It's the Twenty-First Century!

As a rule, if you're a new cyclist, you should conduct your business with a bike shop in real life instead of buying online for all the reasons I've mentioned above. However, if you live in a bike-shop-deprived region there are Internet shops that will offer you much better service than a department store. The best of these are usually real bike shops that also have an online presence, though online-only shops are getting more and more adept at offering a fulfilling retail experience.

Depreciation

Okay, you don't have any local bike shops, you don't have the Internet, and your carrier pigeon is simply not strong enough to fly across three states and return with a bike. Fine. Well, before you buy a *new* department store bike, you should at least try for a *used* department store bike. These things are all over the place, so there's not much reason to pay a premium for a new one.

Chapter 2

UNDER-STANDING YOUR BIKE

O kay, the hard part is over. You've got a bike. Now all you have to do is ride it, right?

Not so fast!

The typical driver has no idea what's going on under the hood of their car. Actually, the typical driver doesn't even know how to open the hood.

The beauty of the bicycle, however, is that its simplicity allows you to be more or less completely self-sufficient. So before you take to the roads, bike lanes, multiuse paths, and trails, let's take a little time to understand your bike so you don't wind up stranded with it.

WHAT IS YOUR BIKE MADE FROM?

We're not going to get into metallurgy here. First, I was an English major. Second, if you got your bike from a reputable bike shop you've almost certainly got a well-designed frame. When a frame has been designed well, it almost doesn't matter what it's made from, so long as it's not ice or chocolate.

If you go through normal, non-big-box channels it's pretty hard to buy a genuinely lousy bike.

(If you bought your bike used or from a store that sells lawn furniture, or you rescued one from a garage, then yes, it is possible you've got a lousy bike. But don't worry. Realizing you've got a lousy bike is an important milestone, because it means you've learned enough to discern its lousiness. Until then, just ride the thing and don't worry about it, and replace it only if and when its lousiness becomes apparent.)

Still, you should be familiar with your frame material, because (1) it influences how you'll have to care for your bike, and (2) you look silly if someone asks you what your bike's made from and you can't answer.

Here are the most common materials used for making bikes.

Steel

There are lots of different types of steels used to make bikes, from the expensive stuff the artisan frame builders use to the relatively cheap stuff mass-market manufacturers employ to make utility bikes.

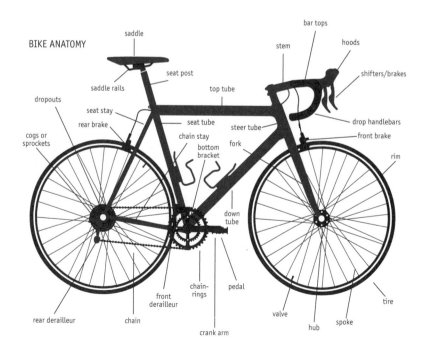

BIKE ANATOMY

Among the self-ordained cycling cognoscenti, steel has a reputation for providing a magical ride that can only be expressed in pretentious contradictions: laterally stiff yet vertically compliant, firm yet supple, stiff yet yielding, and so forth.

Mostly, steel has acquired all this romance because it's traditionally what almost all bikes were made from in the first place, so it's only natural that nostalgia would ascribe to it a certain mystique. Really, these fantastical attributes can be attributed to the ethereal nature of cycling itself. There are few sensations more pleasant than riding a bike. As far as actual magic, the most magical thing about steel is that magnets stick to it.

Nevertheless, steel is indeed a truly excellent material for bikes, mostly because you don't have to be very careful with it. Generally speaking, steel can bend a lot before it breaks, which means if you drop the bike and it gets dented you usually don't have to worry that the frame is now compromised structurally and will fail underneath you when you least expect it. It also means that, if you're constantly locking your bike to crowded bike racks, any damage your bike sustains is likely to be cosmetic.

On the downside, it's true that steel rusts, but unless you leave your bike chained to a boardwalk, exposed to salty sea air day after day for a period of years, it's not going to be a problem. If you insist on worrying anyway, you can treat the inside of the frame with a rust inhibitor sold specifically for that purpose.

The bottom line is that steel is like the denim of frame materials: It can be fancy or it can be practical, but it's pretty difficult to screw it up.

Aluminum

There's a persistent myth among cyclists that aluminum produces a "rougher" ride than other materials. This is nonsense. It may have been true decades ago when aluminum bike frames were still relatively rare and, therefore, unrefined, but bike builders have long since figured out how to use aluminum well. If comfort is a concern for you, there is no reason to avoid a modern aluminum bike.

The chief advantages of aluminum over steel are that it tends to be lighter, it doesn't rust, and manufacturers can form the tubing into all sorts of wacky shapes. (Think aerodynamic time-trial bikes, for example.)

The chief disadvantage is mostly aesthetic. Aluminum frames use larger diameter tubing. Therefore, steel frames look more "traditional," while shaped aluminum frames can look either excitingly modern or offensively clunky, depending on your sensibility. So, while aluminum is a great material for bicycles (especially performance bicycles where weight and aerodynamics are key), it lacks steel's cachet. After all, steel is used to make swords; aluminum is used to make sandwich wrapping.

Carbon Fiber

Carbon fiber has pretty much taken over the high-performance bicycle market. It's light. It's strong. Because it's basically just fabric impregnated with resin, bike builders can mold it into pretty much any shape they want. It also gets people very excited, because while steel and aluminum are all around us, carbon fiber is still relatively exotic. When was the last time you wrapped your sandwich in carbon fiber?

Unfortunately, carbon fiber also has some drawbacks for regular nonsponsored riders, which many people blinded by the performance aesthetic tend to ignore. The chief drawbacks of carbon fiber are:

- It is expensive relative to steel and aluminum.
- It is extremely difficult to recycle, so no smugness for you.
- It is far more likely to be destroyed in crashes and other mishaps.

That last one is significant. Carbon fiber bikes are very strong, provided you use them exactly the way they were designed to be used—that is to say, riding them quickly. If, however, you crash, a carbon fiber bike may be less likely to survive than a metal one. The same goes for less catastrophic, more common cycling mishaps, such as dropping the bike, overtightening a bolt, or forgetting to take the bike off the roof rack before driving into the garage.

(Broken carbon fiber can be repaired, though it will cost you, and damage caused by crashes or general ham-handedness are not covered under most warranties.)

Of course, nobody likes to think about that stuff when buying a bike, which is why carbon fiber has become the default performance material and everything else is increasingly seen as a budget alternative. The truth is that a metal bike will offer all the performance of a carbon fiber one, plus it will provide you with a wider margin for error—and best of all, it will be cheaper, leaving you with more money left over for race registration fees.

Oh, what's that? You don't race? *So what the heck do you need a carbon fiber bike for?*

All of this is to say that if your bicycle is made from carbon fiber, don't crash.

Titanium

Titanium bikes appeal to traditionalists because they are made from metal and look like classic bikes, but they have the dual advantage of being both lighter and more expensive than steel so you can lord your superiority over pretty much everybody. Titanium is also very strong, and unlike steel, you can leave titanium unpainted and it won't rust.

Why leave your fancy high-end bike naked instead of painting it a cool color?

So everyone knows it's titanium, silly!

Bamboo

Yes, people are making bikes out of bamboo now. Why? As bamboo enthusiasts point out, not only is the material extremely strong, but it's also a renewable resource, which makes it environmentally friendly. (I'm not sure this makes much difference since the rest of the bike is made from the usual assortment of metal, rubber, and plastic, but "going green" doesn't always hold up to close scrutiny, does it?)

Most bamboo bikes come from boutique builders, so chances are you aren't going to walk into your local bike shop and walk out with a bamboo bike. However, there are workshops where they'll help you build one for yourself, which may appeal to you if you want to tell people at the café that you made your own bike, or if you're one of those people who has a composting toilet or converted your Volkswagen to run on french fry grease.

As far as caring for your bamboo bike, by far the most important thing to remember is not to leave it near a hungry panda.

STORING YOUR BIKE

Your baby's home. You know what it's made from. And now you're beaming, like a proud parent—but then panic sets in. What now? How do I store it? What if it gets wet? If I hang it by the wheels will it explode?

Relax. The first thing you need to know is that it's a bike, and bikes are tough. You can baby this thing all you want, but rest assured you don't have to. Your bike can handle anything you throw at it.*

Still, you've got a nestling here, so you need to exercise reasonable care. First, find a safe place for your bike to sleep, either outside or inside.

Outside

If your bike is going to live outside, I'm assuming either you're desperate or else you've gone out of your way to purchase a bicycle that can live *al fresco*, and that it has internal gearing and an enclosed drivetrain that are protected from the elements (like

* The author assumes you are not strong enough to throw a washing machine at your bike, because your bike can't handle that.

a typical Dutch bike, for example). You might be able to get away with keeping your minimalist one-speed faux-messenger city bike outside, but if you store a finely tuned bike with exposed derailleurs and gears outdoors for any length of time, the performance will degrade quickly. It's not worth it.

Assuming your bike can withstand the elements, theft is the biggest danger it faces living outside, but a close second is cars. The sidewalks and lampposts of big cities are lined with the twisted carcasses of bicycles that have fallen victim to inept parallel parkers. Park the bike as far from the curb as possible.

You should also cover your saddle. Don't get too fancy about it, a plastic bag will work fine—unless you live in a city like Portland where they hate plastic bags and using one will likely get you pelted with artisanal pickles. If you've got a leather saddle, it's essential to keep it dry or else it will become misshapen and fall apart like an old shoe. However, even if your saddle is waterproof plastic, you should cover it, because sooner or later a bird is going to relieve itself there and you're not going to notice it until you get to work and your co-worker who does triathlons points out that your pants are soiled.

Also, check for "No Parking" (or "No Bikes") signs! You probably do this as a matter of course when you're driving (in this case, they'd be "No Parking" signs), but you may be under the impression that bikes are different and you can leave them anywhere. This is not necessarily the case. You never know when you're going to fall victim to some city employee or a building superintendent with an angle grinder and an unwavering dedication to keeping the front gate bike free.

If you have snowy winters where you live, try to park your bike someplace where snowbanks don't accumulate. Otherwise it will get buried, you'll think it was stolen, and when the thaw finally comes you'll be surprised to find a rusted skeleton in the shape of your bike.

Most important, don't obstruct pathways, doorways, or stairs with your bicycle, because anybody who falls over it is well within their rights to deflate your tires, leave chewed gum on your saddle, or otherwise sabotage your bike.

I know I would.

Inside

Okay, you don't have a Dutch bike or a bakfiets. You've got some kind of sporting bike, and therefore you need to keep it inside some kind of structure that has a ceiling, walls, and a floor.

If it's possible to keep your bicycle inside your climate-controlled home, then great, but if it has to live inside a basement, shed, or garage that's fine too. You may hear horror stories about tires dry rotting, carbon fiber delaminating, and drivetrains seizing irrevocably as a consequence of basement storage, but none of this is really a factor as long as you take reasonable care and use the bike regularly. (And as long as your basement isn't prone to flooding.)

So no, you don't need to run out and purchase a space heater, dehumidifier, and baby monitor for your bike. However, if you are using some kind of common storage area, such as an apartment building bike room, be aware that your neighbors may be inconsiderate types who jam their bikes in next to yours and get their pedals all tangled up in your spokes. So if you share a storage space, use a rack or a hook or other means of hoisting or otherwise segregating your bike if at all possible.

Also, if you keep your bike in a storage area as opposed to inside your home where you see it every day, you should always use a bike lock, because bike room and basement thefts are at least as common as street thefts.

Don't rely on locked doors. If someone wants in, they're getting in.

As for storing your bike inside your actual living space, this allows you to keep close tabs on it; plus, it affords you plenty of opportunity to study, admire, maintain, and otherwise lavish attention upon your beloved bicycle. However, it is also a sign that you are a giant bike dork, so if you share your living space with other humans who do not share your enthusiasm for velocipedes, cohabitation with your bike may or may not place undue strain on the relationship. Know your partner! Some noncyclists are fine with having bikes in the house, while others consider it only slightly better than allowing friends to couch surf for months on end.

Of course, you can always optimize your indoor bicycle storage with some sort of decorative rack or other solution, but keep in mind that these things can cause more problems than they solve. Not only do some of these racks take up space in and of themselves, but they're also more permanent, and sometimes it's better to just lean your bike against a wall so when someone yells, "Get that damn bike out of here!" all you have to do is wheel it into another room.

And no, hanging your bike by the wheels won't hurt the wheels or anything else on the bike—just as long as you've mounted the

Places to keep your bike

- **THE FOYER**
  Good: Doesn't take up actual living space
  Bad: Visitors may trip over it

- **THE KITCHEN**
  Good: Easy cleanup
  Bad: Midnight snacking mishaps

- **THE LIVING ROOM**
  Good: Looks urban like the *Seinfeld* set
  Bad: You may be tempted to perform maintenance during movie night

- **THE BATHROOM**
  Good: Makes a great towel rack
  Bad: Too much humidity

- **THE BEDROOM**
  Good: It's the last thing you see before you go to sleep
  Bad: You don't see it at all when you get up in the middle of the night, so you fall over it

hook to the wall properly. If you haven't, it could fall on your head and kill you.

Most important: *Get insurance!* You should already have homeowner's or renter's insurance. If you don't, get it. Either way, make sure your bicycle is covered. Also, sometimes your policy will cover theft from places other than your home. Consult your insurer.

INDOOR RACKING SYSTEMS

There are all kinds of hardware to help you store your bike inside. Some hardware is unobtrusive, and some is as bulky as home gym equipment. Here are some of the most popular.

WALL HOOK

Pros:

✔ It doesn't take up much space on the wall.

✔ It keeps the bike off the floor and safe from babies, pets, and your Roomba.

Cons:

✘ You have to drill it into your walls.

✘ Your bike is perpendicular to the wall and therefore juts into the room, taking up space.

✘ You have to lift the bike on and off the hook, so if your bike is heavy, it might not be worth the hassle, especially after a long ride when hoisting your bike is the last thing you want to do.

CEILING-MOUNTED HOISTS AND PULLEY SYSTEMS

Pros:

✔ They're perfect for your garage or other lofty storage space.

Cons:

✘ They require high ceilings.

✘ You have to raise and lower your bike whenever you want to ride it, like you're a stagehand and the ride is a production of *Faust* at the Metropolitan Opera.

FLOOR STANDS

Pros:

✔ They're nonpermanent.

✔ There're no more scuffs on the wall from leaning your bike against it.

✔ You can wheel your bike in and out of it, as easy as can be.

Cons:

✗ Your bike takes up precious floor space.

FREESTANDING STORAGE RACKS

Pros:

✔ They're nonpermanent.

✔ Your bike is parallel with the wall so you're less likely to walk into it.

✔ You can store two or more bikes at a time, one on top of the other.

Cons:

✗ They're somewhat bulky and ugly, so best relegated to the basement.

ESSENTIAL REPAIRS AND MAINTENANCE YOU SHOULD KNOW
Roadside Repairs
FLATS

One of the greatest attributes of the bicycle is simplicity. It takes only a little bit of competency to ensure you never get stranded, and by far the most common scenario for getting stranded is the flat tire.

Your tires are the most vulnerable component of your bicycle. It is a truism of cycling that punctures happen. When they do, you're stuck. It's another truism of cycling that you're either inexcusably lazy or irredeemably foolish if you don't at least take an afternoon and learn how to fix a flat. In a perfect world, you wouldn't even be *allowed* to ride a bicycle until you demonstrated your ability to repair your own tire.

For a detailed seminar on fixing a flat there are hundreds of flat repair instructional videos on YouTube. I implore you to *watch them!* (Not all of them, of course, but at least a few.) And don't stop there. Read some old-fashioned how-to articles while you're at it, because pro mechanics can convey nuances that instructional videos cannot.

Once you've consumed this information, *try it yourself with your own bicycle.* Remove your wheel from your bike, then remove the tire from the wheel, then remove the tube, replace it, and put the whole thing back together again. Do it with the front wheel, then do it with the back wheel. If you don't have all the tools you need to do this, *go buy those tools!* Remember when I told you not to leave the bike shop without everything you need to fix a flat? If you did anyway, now's the time to correct that.

Learn all the quirks and particulars of your bike's setup in the comfort of your own home, because you don't want to have to do it for the first time by the side of the road when darkness is falling and so is the temperature. For example, depending on your setup, you may need to remove a rack or fender struts in order to get the wheel out. Find out now, not later!

Once you venture out for your first ride, and every single ride thereafter, *make sure you have everything with you to fix a flat.* This means both the know-how and the tools. Unless mountain lions have torn your tires apart, there's no excuse for getting stranded because of a flat.

Finally, and I can't stress this enough, *always carry a pump.* Carry CO_2 inflators if you must, but only if you have a pump as a backup. A CO_2 cartridge is great for bringing your tire up to full pressure in a matter of seconds, but it is of no use to you when you screw up with the inflator and it expels itself prematurely.

There are two basic types of portable bicycle pump:

1. Frame pump. This type of pump gets wedged into your frame, usually between the head tube and the seat tube, and it stays

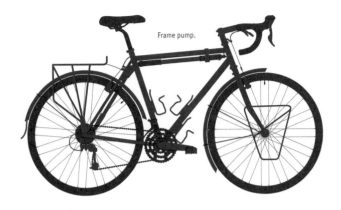

Frame pump.

there by means of spring tension, like a shower caddy you'd find at Bed Bath & Beyond.

The advantage of the frame pump is that you can bring your tire up to full pressure relatively easily. The disadvantage is that it takes up some real estate on your bike, and not all frames can accommodate one.

2. Mini pump. These range from small to teensy-weensy, and you can either stick it in your pocket or bag or else mount it behind your water bottle cage.

The advantage of the mini pump is its extreme portability. The disadvantage is that, while it will certainly get you going again, it may be difficult or impossible to get your tire up to full pressure with one. Plus, if you've got a high-volume tire (as you'd find on a mountain bike, for example), you will be pumping furiously for a prolonged period of time.

Mini pump.

By the way, lots of bike shops offer classes that teach you basic skills like fixing a flat, so if yours does, you should take advantage of it. Not only will you learn something, but you might meet somebody, fall in love, and live happily ever after, just like in a rom-com.

This is why we like bike shops.

||||||||||||||||||||

PATCHING TUBES AND BOOTING TIRES

• PATCHING TUBES

Throwing away an inner tube after a single puncture is like throwing out your socks after wearing them once. Don't ditch your tube after changing it. That's wasteful. Patch it instead.

A correctly installed patch isn't a temporary solution. Once you've patched a tube, you can keep riding and forget about it. Just make sure you follow the directions on the package.

You can patch your tube more than once. It's perfectly fine to repair a tube multiple times, as long as the patches don't overlap.

• BOOTING A TIRE

If your tire falls victim to a gash so severe that the casing is compromised and the tube is exposed, you can still get home by "booting" the tire. Fold up a dollar bill, energy bar wrapper, or something similarly strong yet flexible and place it on the *inside* of the tire so

it covers the entire cut. Make sure the edges of the boot lie smoothly between the inside of the tire and the tube, then remount the tire and inflate. Also make sure to replace the tire before your next ride. (And retrieve your money, of course.)

• MAINTAINING TUBES

Check your spare tubes from time to time. A tube that's been living in a saddlebag for years can eventually wear through or fall victim to dry rot, and you won't notice it until you're stranded with a flat on the side of the road. To maximize your spare tube's life, you can keep it in a sandwich bag. Also, keep the valve cap on; otherwise the valve stem can wear a hole in the tube.

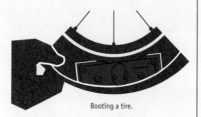

Booting a tire.

PRO TIP

Finding the piece of debris that caused your puncture can be tricky, but there's a way to make it easier. Your tire's sidewall has a brand label. When installing your tire, align that label with your valve stem. Then, when you get a flat, find the hole in the tube in relation to the valve stem. Because your label is always aligned with your valve stem, you now know approximately where on the tire the piece of debris that caused the puncture must have entered.

DRIVETRAIN ISSUES

While your chain and gears might stop working properly during your ride, it's pretty unlikely they'll actually fail completely and stop you altogether. Usually what happens is the bike stops shifting properly, in which case you pick a gear that works and fix the problem when you get home.

Many bicycles and pretty much all "sporting" ones shift by means of derailleurs, which are those mechanisms that move the chain from one sprocket to another.

Derailleurs are often intimidating to the novice, but they're actually pretty simple, and the fact that they're completely exposed makes them easy to study and work on.

Assuming you have a derailleur drivetrain, if anything's going to bring you to a halt it's your chain falling off the chainring, which can happen if your system is out of adjustment or you pedal through bumpy terrain when your chain happens to be in a gear combo that results in a lot of slack. We call this "dropping your chain." While the experienced cyclist can often finesse a dropped chain back onto the chainring while riding, if you are not an experienced cyclist, do not attempt this. Instead, *stop the bike immediately*. If you keep pedaling you're only going to make it worse because the

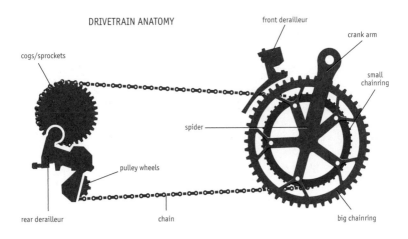

DRIVETRAIN ANATOMY

front derailleur

crank arm

cogs/sprockets

small chainring

spider

pulley wheels

rear derailleur   chain   big chainring

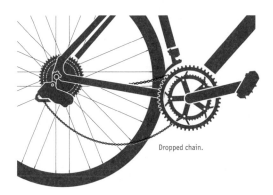

Dropped chain.

chain can jam, and in the worst case, you might damage the chain, the derailleur, or even the frame.

Okay. You've stopped. The chain is hanging off your bike like toilet paper off a suburban tree on Halloween night. First, shift your front derailleur to the smallest chainring if it's not there already. Next, lean down and push the rear derailleur with your left hand toward the front of the bike to create slack in the chain. Then lift the chain with your right hand. (*Yes, with your hand.* I know it's dirty but deal with it.) Now wrap it around the smallest chainring. Once it's where it's supposed to be, let the derailleur go, pick up the rear wheel, and turn the pedal by hand to make sure the chain is running smoothly before getting back on the bike.

If it's a particularly bad chain derailment, the chain may have made its way off the rear derailleur pulleys too. This can be vexing,

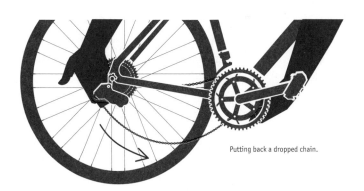

Putting back a dropped chain.

and in fact you may not be able to figure out how it even got like that in the first place. When dealing with a severe chain derailment the key is *don't panic.* Take your time. Study the problem. Figure out how to extricate and realign everything, and do so gingerly.

Your hands will get filthy, but you'll get it sorted eventually.

In the worst case, you may find that your chain has broken. This rare scenario is scarier than it sounds, and fixing a chain really isn't that difficult, although it does require using a chain tool. Here's where those online instructional videos on fixing a chain will come in handy again. It's also useful to find an old piece of bike chain and practice on that by breaking it and reconnecting it a few times.

However, chains break so infrequently that you generally shouldn't have to worry about carrying a chain tool around with you. It's more of a concern when mountain biking, where mud, branches, and other forms of debris are more likely to snarl, jam, or otherwise contaminate your drivetrain, so think about adding a small portable chain tool to your pack if you're doing any big off-road rides.

Assuming you have a chain tool and you know how to use it, all you have to do in the event of a broken chain is remove the damaged link, thereby shortening the chain slightly. This may mean you'll have some unusable gear combinations now, so be careful when you shift, but at least you'll get home.

POST-CRASH OR MISHAP, INSPECTION, AND ADJUSTMENT

Remember I said you should always carry a multitool? This is why.

So you've fallen off your bike for one reason or another. It's okay. It's happened to all of us. Once you've established that you're okay, you should move on to inspecting the bike, because you don't want to get back on only to discover something's wrong when it breaks and you fall right back off again.

You may find that your saddle and handlebars are twisted. If they are, don't attempt to twist them back by hand. If you've watched the Tour de France, you've probably seen a crashed rider leap to his feet and pound the nose of his saddle until it's straight again. This is not a good idea, because it's entirely possible yours will simply break and fly right off your bike. The same thing goes for your handlebars. Don't hold your front wheel between your knees and twist, especially if you've got a carbon fiber fork. Carbon fiber doesn't like that.

Instead, take your multitool—*you know, the one you always carry with you*—and re-align everything. Once everything is back where it belongs, grab your brakes and rock the bike back and forth. Not only will this tell you if the brakes are working, but if your carbon steerer tube is broken, you want your handlebars to fall off now as opposed to when you start riding again.

Repairing a wheel on the fly

If you're *really* far from home, your wheel is *really* out of true, and it's either get it rolling again or walk for three hours (and you happen to have a spoke wrench on you, which you probably don't), here's how you do it:

1. Turn your bike upside down.
2. Spin the wheel.
3. Observe where it gets stuck.
4. Look at the rim at that spot. Now, find the pair of spokes closest to that spot that run to the *opposite side of the hub* from the side of the wheel that's stuck.
5. Tighten both spoke nipples until that spot is no longer stuck and the rim is closer to the center line of the frame. (Spokes are right-hand threaded, which means that technically righty-tighty, lefty-loosey applies. However, when the bike is upside down and you tighten a spoke nipple on a wheel that's already assembled, you are in effect turning it *counterclockwise*, because you're essentially looking at the underside of the nipple. The actual head of the nipple is underneath the tire and the rim tape.)
6. If it's getting hard to turn the spoke nipples, find the pair of spokes closest to that spot that run to the *same side of the hub as where the wheel is stuck* and *loosen* the nipples.

Even if the wheel is wobbly because you broke a spoke, you can still use this method to tweak the wheel so that it's rideable, but be careful how much you tighten the remaining spokes, because if you overdo it you can strip the spoke threads.

Next, lift your bike and spin your wheels, one at a time. Do they turn freely or do they stop? If they stop, why? Did the crash knock them out of the frame? Loosen the quick release, reseat them in the dropouts, and tighten again. Did your brake calipers move? Move them back. (If you've got sidepull calipers, you can usually do this by hand.) Is the wheel wobbly? Open your brake a bit so the wheel can turn yet the brake still works, and then once you get home, true the wheel as soon as you can. Is the wheel *really* wobbly, so much so that it won't even pass through the frame when the brakes are wide open? That's trickier, although with a spoke wrench even a novice can reshape the wheel into something that can roll again.

Wheels can be confusing if not bewildering, and if you want to fully understand the physics behind them you should read *The Bicycle Wheel*, by Jobst Brandt, or at least Sheldon Brown's writing (sheldonbrown.com) on the subject. However, for the purposes of getting home, think of it this way: The spokes are basically strings that pull the rim in the direction you want it to go. Follow the spoke from the rim to the hub and you can figure out which ones to turn to pull the rim. If you're patient and keep this principle in mind, you can at least get yourself rolling again in an emergency.

Finally, if the brakes work, the parts are reasonably straightish, and the bike seems like it will roll, lift it up and drop it again a few times and make sure nothing else falls off. If it doesn't, continue on your way, but do so gingerly lest some unseen problem reveal itself. If it does, figure out what it is and put it back.

Routine Maintenance

Your bicycle doesn't need much in the way of maintenance. You don't need to follow a schedule, you don't need to mind an odometer, and you don't need some silly smartphone app that alerts you to rotate your tires and overhaul your bottom bracket.

Potentially the hardest thing about bike maintenance is saying the word "nipples" without giggling.

If you can do the following things you're at least 90 percent of the way to self-sufficiency in keeping your bike running trouble free.

LUBING YOUR CHAIN

When it comes to keeping your bike in good running order, by far the most important thing you can do on a day-to-day basis is keep the chain lubricated. How often you need to do this depends on how and where you ride, but at the very least do it whenever you hear the beginnings of anything that sounds like chirping or squeaking.

When it comes to drivetrain sounds, some "thrumming" is normal, but tortured rodent cries are not.

Lengthy magazine articles have been written about which lube to use and how to apply it, but it's really not worth thinking too much about. Just get a bicycle-specific chain lube from the bike shop and follow the directions on the bottle. (You don't even have to use bicycle-specific chain lube if you don't want to—oil works fine—but the boutique bike stuff tends to be cleaner, the packaging is convenient, and in the grand scheme of life it's not *that* expensive, so go ahead and treat yourself. You deserve it.)

Don't be afraid of your chain, either. Yes, it's the filthiest part of your bike, and yes, it's all moving parts, but it's a fairly cheap component and it will work for years with minimal attention.

CLEANING YOUR CHAIN

Sadly, cyclists are highly susceptible to drivetrain scare tactics. People who write for bike magazines will tell you that it's vital to keep your chain clean. They'll point to how all that road grit will work its way into the pins and plates and rollers and eat it away from the inside, taking the rest of your components with it.

Nah.

The truth is, if you don't know what you're doing, it's constant cleaning that will *shorten* your chain's life. Various companies sell

||||||||||||||||||||

CLEANING YOUR CHAIN

If your chain has gotten to the point where you feel you must clean it, here's how to do it*:

1. Remove chain. (Take care not to mangle the outer plates. That's why you practiced on an old piece of bike chain, remember?)

2. Put it in a big plastic soda bottle (a clean, empty one, not one filled with soda, silly).

3. Add a solvent such as mineral spirits or Simple Green, replace cap.

4. Shake vigorously. How vigorously? Well, if you've got a dog, it should be barking, and if you've got a cat, it should be hiding under the bed. To be sure you have cleaned the chain thoroughly, dance wildly to "Walking on Sunshine," by Katrina and the Waves, all the way through at least twice.

Note: These chain cleaning instructions apply mostly to sporting bikes with exposed derailleur drivetrains. If you're riding a bike with a chain guard or an enclosed drivetrain, like a Dutch bike, for example, congratulations! Chances are you can pretty much ignore your chain altogether for many years, save for the occasional lubing.

5. Rinse the chain in clean water and dry it.

6. Reinstall chain.

7. Lubricate chain.

8. Dispose of solvent responsibly, or else filter out the grit and save for next time.

PRO TIP

Chains these days come in all different sizes for all the different drivetrain configurations out there, and they also often have proprietary pins and links. After you've removed your chain the first time, do yourself a favor and get one of those reusable "quick links" you can connect and disconnect again and without tools. These come in different widths for different chains, so make sure you get the appropriate one for yours. Once you've installed one of these things, chain removal and reinstallation are only slightly more difficult than putting on jewelry, and you'll only need to deal with a chain tool if you get a new chain and have to size it.

all sorts of plastic machines that purport to clean your chain while it's still on the bike. These appeal to people who like clean bikes but are too afraid to get their hands dirty and remove their chains. However, all these contraptions really do is clean the *outside* of the chain while driving more crap *inside* where the actual wear occurs.

So forget the chain cleaning devices. It's better not to clean your chain at all. When it comes to chain life, lubrication is far more important than cleanliness.

So when *should* you clean your chain? Only when you can't stand how dirty it is. The real problem with a dirty chain is that you can't work on your bike without getting filthy. Removing your wheel or replacing a dropped chain is easy, but it's annoying and inconvenient when you become covered in chain grease in the process, and your noncycling partner will not appreciate your leaving fingerprints all over the house after every ride.

Another hazard of an overly dirty chain is the dreaded "chainring tattoo": the greasy, black imprint of the chainring that mars the back of the leg when you go to straddle the bike and accidentally touch your calf to the chain. It's the cycling equivalent of walking around with toilet paper stuck to your shoe. Not good.

REPLACING YOUR CHAIN

How do you know when you need a new chain? The big tip-off that you need a new chain is if your bike shifts poorly despite your derailleurs being in proper adjustment. However, if you want to get ridiculously technical about it, as a chain wears, the longer it stretches, and at a certain point it gets so long that it will wear out your cogs too. Then you've got to replace your chain *and* your cogs, because your worn cogs won't mesh with a new chain. So there are two ways to approach chain replacement:

1. Ride until your drivetrain is too worn to shift to your satisfaction and then replace your chain and cogs. On one hand, this is the more expensive, but on the other hand, it could be years before you have to even worry about it, so it's up to you.

2. Measure your chain periodically. Chain pins are an inch apart, so if you measure twelve links with a one-foot ruler, everything should line up. If it doesn't, it means your chain is stretched and you can replace it preemptively to avoid cog wear. Unless you're doing massive mileage, or you're riding in extremely foul conditions, changing your chain once or twice a year is probably more than sufficient.

You can buy chain measuring devices specifically for this purpose, but an inch is an inch, so any household measuring implement calibrated for those primitive English units will do.

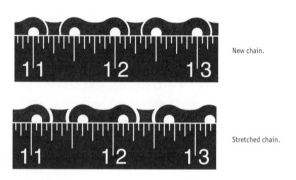

New chain.

Stretched chain.

ADJUSTING YOUR SHIFTING AND GEARS

If you have a bike with an internally geared hub, then congratulations, you will rarely have to think about adjusting it. Usually you can ride and ride for years without much concern. And if it does start misbehaving, it's probably a simple matter of turning a single screw or adjuster somewhere. Just look at the brand and model name of your hub, search for it on the Internet, and follow the directions for adjustment. It's often as easy as that.

Derailleurs are a bit more sensitive, but they're also very simple to adjust once you understand how they work.

Keeping your derailleurs in adjustment is very much like tuning a guitar. The barrel adjusters are the tuning pegs, the cables are the strings, and your bicycle is the guitar. It's all a matter of getting the tension right. If the bike's in tune, it will shift cleanly and crisply. If it's out of tune, it will chatter and rattle.

The key is in knowing which way to turn those damn barrel adjusters. If you turn all your guitar tuning pegs willy-nilly, you'll soon be completely lost sonically. If, however, you understand which peg controls which string, and that tightening them raises the pitch and loosening them lowers it, then you can quickly make sense of the procedure. As it happens, a bike's much easier, since there are only the two derailleurs to worry about. It's like tuning a two-stringed guitar.

REAR SHIFTING

Your derailleur is a spring. When that spring is unloaded and re-laxed, the rear derailleur is sitting over your smallest cog, which is your "fastest" or "hardest" gear.

Your shifter works by pulling your derailleur, which in turn nudges the chain onto a bigger cog (or "easier" gear). Imagine walking a dog up a staircase. If you're having trouble shifting from a harder gear into an easier gear, adjust the derailleur by turning the barrel adjuster incrementally, toward the bike to tighten the cable until the bike is shifting smoothly. (If you look closely, you'll

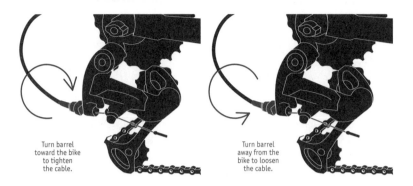

Turn barrel
toward the bike
to tighten
the cable.

Turn barrel
away from the
bike to loosen
the cable.

notice your barrel adjuster has notches or detents in it; turn it one notch at a time.)

When you shift into a smaller cog (or "harder" gear), your shifter is releasing the cable just enough to allow the derailleur to move down one gear. If your bike is shifting poorly from an easy gear to a harder gear, you'll need to adjust the derailleur by turning the barrel away from the bike and loosening the cable very slowly until it does, so the dog can walk back down the steps.

FRONT SHIFTING

When your front derailleur is relaxing, it's hunkering down next to your seat tube with the chain around the little ring. So when you shift to the big ring, the cable's pulling the front derailleur up and away from the frame, and together with the chainring teeth, it has to hoist the chain from the smaller chainring to the larger one.

This is a big job for a derailleur, which is why the front upshift is often the most trouble-prone one.

If, when you try to shift, all you hear is a bunch of clattering as the chain tries and fails to grab the big chainring, the cable needs to be tighter.

So tighten it by turning the barrel adjuster counterclockwise, as with your rear derailleur.

When you shift back into the smaller ring, you're releasing that cable tension. This allows the derailleur to return to its resting position, taking the chain with it. If there's too much tension in the cable, that won't happen, because the derailleur won't return all the way. Loosen the cable until there's no tension on the derailleur in the resting position, but not so much that there's actual slack in the cable.

Note: Depending on your bike, your front derailleur cable may or may not have a barrel adjuster. If it does, you will probably find it either on the shifter cable stop on your downtube or else near the shifter along the shifter cable itself. If it doesn't, you need to loosen the cable anchor bolt (this is the bolt that cinches the cable to the derailleur), pull the cable taut, and refasten.

THROWING THE CHAIN

Your front and rear derailleurs have screws that determine how far they are allowed to move in either direction. If these parameters are too narrow, you can't use all your gear combinations. If they're too wide, you can shift the chain right off the chainrings, or you can shift your rear derailleur right past your biggest cog and into your spokes, ruining your derailleur, wheel, and possibly even your frame in the process. This is known as the bike "throwing its chain."

Each derailleur has two screws: the outer-limit screw and the inner-limit screw. They're a teeny set of Phillips-head screws, and if you look closely you can even see where they stop the derailleur from moving past a certain point. To understand how they work,

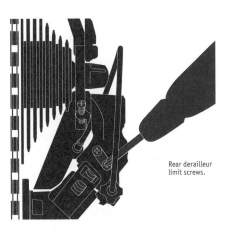

Rear derailleur limit screws.

take the chain off your bike, get in really close, and push the derailleur with your hand. Taking ten or fifteen minutes to study how your derailleur works is worth it, and while your hands might get a little dirty, it's a lot more informative than reading a PDF of the instruction manual.

If your bike is throwing its chain past the gears when you shift, *check these screws*. They should be set so that your derailleurs absolutely *cannot move* past the inner and outer cogs and chainrings.

To check, shift into the troublesome gear combinations while you're off the bike. Then nudge the shifter and see if the derailleur continues to move. If it does, close the limit screw until it doesn't anymore.

Don't ride the bike again until you're satisfied that it's impossible to shift the chain off the gears.

MAINTAINING AND REPLACING YOUR TIRES
Your life depends on the integrity of your tires, so inspect them regularly for:

- Cuts
- Cracks
- Tread wear

None of these issues necessarily mean you need to change your tires.

Sure, your coworker who does triathlons will faint at the sight of your blemished rubber, but we live in disposable times, and often we're way too quick to throw away perfectly good tires.

A little cosmetic cracking in your tire's tread is usually just that. Moreover, over time, grit and gravel and little bits of wire and tiny shards of glass will leave cuts and holes in your tire here and there. This is normal. If tire tread wasn't soft enough to yield to debris now and again, your bike would have all the cornering traction of a shopping cart.

Even tread wear isn't such a big deal unless you can see the casing of the tire. (That's the woven layer of nylon or cotton that

When should you replace a tire?

• WORN RUBBER

Would you wear a sneaker without a sole? No, you wouldn't. So don't ride a tire worn to the casing.

• DEEP CUTS

There's a difference between a paper cut and a machete wound. One hurts if you get lemon juice on it, and the other will cause you to bleed out in short order. The same goes for your tires. A small cut here and there is no big deal, but the casing is what's holding your tire together, so when it's compromised your tire becomes a liability. Any cut that goes through the casing of your tire is a reason for concern. If you can see inner tube through a cut when your tire is inflated, then it's time for a new tire.

• SUSPICIOUS BULGES

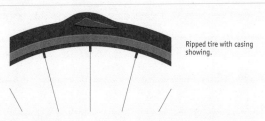

Ripped tire with casing showing.

Tires are not always perfectly round, as you'll see if you hold your wheel up and spin it. There's usually a visible wobble, but a serious bulge could mean your casing is damaged. Once your casing is damaged, your tire is like Led Zeppelin in the final days of John Bonham—doomed.

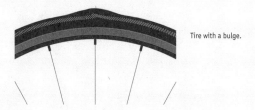

Tire with a bulge.

NOTE: A bulge in your tire could also mean you installed it incorrectly, so inspect and reinstall before declaring it dead.

gives the tire its shape when it's filled with air.) Sure, it's prudent to replace a tire before it gets to that point, but there's no big hurry either. If you look at the profile of your tire and it's drastically squared off instead of rounded, then you may want to start thinking about tire replacement, but the situation isn't truly urgent until that casing starts peeking out at you.

Also, keep in mind that your tire's tread pattern is generally a poor gauge of tire wear. Just because the little indentations are disappearing doesn't mean your traction is too. If you ride a road or pavement-oriented bike, your tire's tread is mostly cosmetic. Of course it's a different story with knobby tires, because if you ride in the dirt, those knobs are actually doing something. So when the knobs are gone, replace the tire—and if your knobbies wear out really quickly because you only use them on pavement, *stop wasting tires by riding knobbies* on the road. You might as well walk around in soccer cleats.

TIRE ROTATION

Not only is your bicycle rear-wheel drive, but most of your weight is directly over that rear wheel as well. Therefore, your rear tire will wear out well before your front.

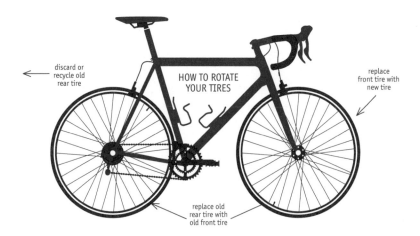

discard or recycle old rear tire

HOW TO ROTATE YOUR TIRES

replace front tire with new tire

replace old rear tire with old front tire

It's not uncommon for a tire to die prematurely due to glass and other debris, but if you're fortunate enough to see a rear tire through to the end of its life, remove it and buy *one* new tire. Move your current front tire to the rear wheel and put the new tire on the front wheel.

Repeat this cycle for the life of your bicycle. It will maximize the life of your tires and save you money.

When it comes to tires, think of your bicycle as a living thing, like a snake shedding its own skin, or some kind of lizard that eats and excretes tires. Food goes in front, excrement goes out the back. Not the other way around.

BIKE FIT, ADJUSTMENTS, AND UPGRADES

Now that you understand how your bike works, it's time to get to know each other more intimately, so light some candles and cue up the John Mayer.

The first step in this process is dialing in the fit.

If you bought your bike at the pro shop and you sprang for the special bike fitting with the umlauts in its name where they hooked electrodes to your body and pointed lasers at you, just leave your bike the way it is.

Not that I believe deeply in the umlaut method, but hey, if you paid all that money, who am I to tell you to change anything?

Otherwise, spend your first few rides making adjustments to your bicycle. Take your time. Keep your multitool handy. Stop frequently. Experiment. If something feels uncomfortable, go ahead and change it. Tinker with your saddle position and height. Rotate your bars up and down a bit as you see fit. Trust yourself. Worry less about how everything is "supposed" to be and more about what feels good to you right now.

Remember, when you're fine-tuning your bike's fit, it's perfectly fine to play it by ear—or, more accurately, by crotch.

Not only will this make you more comfortable, but it will also familiarize you with the workings of the various fittings of your bicycle.

Just make sure to go easy on those bolts. Today's bicycle fasteners don't require much torque, and it's far easier to overtighten them than it is to undertighten them, especially when it comes to stems and seat post clamps. If you're tightening a small bolt more than you would the cap on a bottle of Snapple, you're probably turning it too hard.

Tuning the Ride

Your bicycle's ride quality is not determined by its frame material— at least not in a significant way. It is determined mainly by:

- Tire width and pressure
- The "contact points" between you and the bike (mainly your saddle and handlebars)
- The geometry of your frame (the wheelbase, the offset of the fork, where the rear wheel is in relation to your backside, etc.)

Of these, tire width and pressure are probably the most important. Lots of new riders (as well as plenty of longtime cyclists) are riding around with too much air in their tires. This is because there's a common misconception that hard tires equal fast bike!

Alas, hard tires do *not* equal fast bike; they equal numb hands and sore arse!

Bike companies, reviewers, and Internet blowhards will also tell you that a frame made out of *x* is "smoother" than a frame made out of *y*. This is ridiculous. They're telling you some infinitesimal difference in resonant frequencies is the difference between comfort and discomfort. Meanwhile here you are rolling on a cushion of air! *And that's* the key to your bike's ride quality. So work with that air cushion! Want a "smoother" ride? Make the cushion softer by letting some of the air out of the tires. Want a "stiffer, more responsive" bike? Put some of that air back in!

If you've ever used an inflatable neck pillow on an airplane you've got the idea.

Remember, there's no "correct" air pressure. Don't go by what it says on your tire's sidewall—that's usually just the *maximum* pressure, which you would never use anyway.

Of course, while you don't want too much air in your tires, you don't want too little in there either. So how do you know if your air pressure is too low?

- Your rims are bottoming out (in other words, your tires are so squishy you can feel the rim hitting the ground from time to time).
- Your tires are squirming underneath you in a disconcerting way when you corner.
- You generally feel like you're riding through Jell-O.

The first two are dangerous; the third one is just annoying.

If you feel like you can't find the sweet spot between "pressure too low" and "teeth rattling out of your head," get wider tires. Volume is good. Not only does more volume usually mean better traction, but the wider your tires are, the less air pressure you need in them. Thirty pounds per square inch is basically a flat tire on a skinny road bike tire where typical pressure generally hovers somewhere in the vicinity of one hundred pounds per square inch, yet it's borderline high on a fat mountain bike tire.

Your grips or bar tape is also highly effective in changing the character of your ride. Some people buy expensive carbon fiber handlebars because they think they will soak up road vibrations better than aluminum ones. This is nonsense. Why do that when all you need is softer grips or cushier bar tape—or even just a pair of padded gloves, for that matter? Grips and bar tape are cheap and easy to install, so experiment and find the one you like best. You may want to change to a different handlebar *shape* if you can't get your hands where you want them, but when it comes to the smoothness of your ride, the material of your bars makes no difference.

As for your frame's geometry, there's not much changing that—the angles that make up your bike are basically its DNA—though

||||||||||||||||||||||

FRAME GEOMETRY ATTRIBUTES YOU MIGHT ACTUALLY NOTICE

Drop the *Princess and the Pea* act. Most riders don't notice frame angle differences of a few degrees. But if you're comparing two similar bikes and find yourself delving into the nitty-gritty of frame geometry, here are the measurements that make the most difference.

• WHEELBASE

The longer the wheelbase, the more "stable" the bike will feel. The bike may also feel "smoother," since you're not sitting directly on top of your rear wheel.

• BOTTOM BRACKET HEIGHT

A lower bottom bracket height means a lower center of gravity, which may enhance feelings of sta-

bility, especially when descending. On the other hand, higher bottom bracket means better ground clearance, which is useful for off-road cycling when you're riding over obstacles, or if you're a track, criterium, or cyclocross racer and you need to pedal through turns.

• HEADTUBE ANGLE

The headtube angle determines your bicycle's "steering axis." Together with fork *rake* (that's how far ahead of the steering axis the fork places the front axle) and *trail* (which is how far behind the steering axis your tire makes contact with the ground), this influences how your bike turns. Generally speaking, a steeper headtube angle makes your bike turn more quickly, while a shallower headtube angle might make the bike feel a bit more stable.

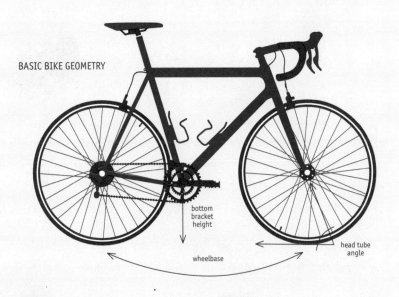

BASIC BIKE GEOMETRY

bottom bracket height

head tube angle

wheelbase

you can change your position on your bike to compensate. Raising or lowering handlebars, moving the saddle fore or aft, and changing the length of your stem can have a significant effect on both comfort and handling.

Wear Items

If you live to upgrade, I've got bad news for you: Bike parts last a really long time. So you're going to need some creative excuses if you want to buy lots of new stuff all the time. (Don't worry, the bike industry and media are always happy to help you with the excuses.)

As for the stuff that does wear out, here's what you should check often and count on having to replace regularly:

• **Brake pads.** No matter what kind of brake calipers you have, they use pads to create friction with the braking surface, and when those pads wear out, the bike doesn't stop anymore and you crash. So check them regularly.

Your rear pads will wear out long before your fronts, so keep that in mind when you're inspecting.

Rim brake pads are right out there in the open, so it's hard not to notice when they're disappearing. Disc brake pads are tucked away inside the caliper, so it's easy to forget about them. Don't. Check them regularly. A well-designed disc brake caliper will have some sort of cutout or window to facilitate inspection.

• **Brake and shifter cables.** Obsessive people replace these once a year, but that's usually not necessary. Replace your cables when they're visibly rusty or frayed, or when they're seized. You'll know they're seized because they'll be corroded and your brakes or shifters will work poorly, or not at all.

• **Brake and shifter housing.** Your cables live inside a plastic (usually) housing. Replace this if it's cracked or if your cables were badly seized. If the housing is intact, and if you can slide a new cable through it easily, don't bother replacing the housing.

• **Rims.** If your bike has rim brakes, then your rim's sidewall will wear out eventually, because it's also your braking surface. Newer rims often have a wear indicator that will become visible when it's time to retire the rim. Older rims won't, so if your rim's sidewall is deeply scored or noticeably concave, you might want to bring it to the shop for them to check it out. It will take you a long, long time to wear out a rim—unless you ride in exceedingly foul conditions, in which case you might want to think about disc brakes.

Note: If you wear out your rim, you don't need a new wheel. All you need is a new rim. You can keep using your same hub and spokes. Yes, you can reuse the spokes. Don't let anyone tell you otherwise. Of course, some companies will charge you so much for a replacement rim that it might almost be cheaper to buy a new wheel, but that's another story.

• **Rotors.** If your bike has disc brakes, it has rotors. Eventually they'll wear out. When they do, replace them. Inspection is very easy. They're right there in plain sight.

• **Cleats.** If you use clipless pedals, the cleats on the bottoms of your shoes will wear out eventually. Check them from time to time, because when your cleats get worn, your feet can pop out of your pedals at inconvenient moments, such as when you're sprinting, which can result in crashing or sudden and painful crotch-top-tube contact.

Most cleats have wear indicators for your convenience.

• **Grips/bar tape.** Yes. When worn, toss and replace.

• **Tires.** Obviously. We've been through this.

• **Chain and gears.** Eventually, as we discussed.

• **Your helmet.** Most companies and shops will tell you to replace your helmet after three years. I am highly skeptical of this. Your helmet is made from EPS foam. More and more cities are banning EPS foam because it's environmentally unfriendly and floats around in the ocean for a thousand years.

Yet it lasts for only three years when it's on your head?

Come on.

Replace your helmet if you crash on it. Otherwise, the most likely reason you'll want to replace your helmet is because you found a cooler one.

CLEANING YOUR BIKE

People are nuts with the bike cleaning. Nuts, I say! Roadies, for example, treat bikes like they're underwear: wash after every use.

The reality, though, is that bikes are much more like jeans: Generally speaking, people wash them way more than they need to, and unless something really nasty happens, then once in a while is plenty.

The best way to wash your bike is with a garden hose if you have access to one. The pressure is ideal, because it will remove dirt, yet it won't blast lube out of those sensitive places. You can use a gentle detergent or degreaser, but often the water is enough. Hose it down, bounce dry, lube chain. Done.

If you're using anything stronger than a garden hose—like a power washer—don't spray it directly into anything that spins (hubs, bottom bracket), because there's grease in those bearings and you want it to stay there. Just imagine power washing yourself. There are certain places you wouldn't want that stream to go, right? Well, your bike has sensitive parts too.

If you don't have access to a hose, a bucket and a sponge or gentle brush will work too.

Some people wash their bikes in the shower or bathtub, but these people tend to live alone and have more than one cat.

ESSENTIAL TOOLS

With these tools, you should be able to do pretty much everything in this section:

- Complete set of Allen wrenches
- Chain tool
- Spoke wrench
- Tire levers
- Floor pump

If you've got all the following stuff in your saddlebag, on your bike, or in your jersey pocket, there's very little you won't be able to fix:

- Multitool
- Chain tool (sometimes included with mini tool)
- Patch kit
- Spare tube
- Tire levers
- Frame or mini pump
- Spoke wrench

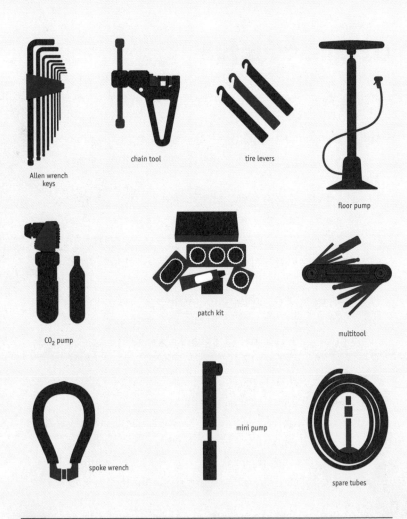

Allen wrench keys

chain tool

tire levers

floor pump

CO_2 pump

patch kit

multitool

spoke wrench

mini pump

spare tubes

I've heard of people who wash bike components in the dishwasher. They live alone and have more than five cats.

In between washes, wipe your bike down with a rag now and again. This will keep the grime in check, but more important, it will help you notice any cracks or other problems you might otherwise easily miss until it's too late.

Most of all, remember: *Dirt won't kill your bike!* Bikes like to be ridden, not washed. A clean bike is a neglected bike.

Chapter 3

PROTECTING AND CARING FOR YOUR BIKE

By now you're probably beginning to form a strong attachment to your bicycle. You gaze lovingly at it. You think about it when you're apart. You may have even assigned it a gender and a name.

Stop right there.

It's normal to bond with and personify inanimate objects, especially when, like bicycles, they play an important role in your life. Plus, bicycles even look kind of mammalian, which is especially endearing. After all, the whole idea of the bicycle is more or less predicated on the horse, and few creatures have a deeper and more profound connection than equines and humans.

But while it's good to have a loving relationship with your two-wheeled steed, you don't want it to go full *Equus*. The more emotion you invest in your bicycle, the more of yourself you're liable to lose if one day it's gone. It's an inconvenient truth that people like to steal bicycles and, what's worse, it's something that's easy to do. Bikes are fast, they're light, they're human powered, they're often left unattended—and the average person can't tell them apart, which makes IDing them difficult. Plus, bikes are pretty much everywhere, wild mulberries ripe for the picking. This means they function as sort of a de facto currency for the criminal underworld, a readily accepted form of illegal tender among the drug-addled and unscrupulous.

PROTECTING YOUR BIKE

It's okay to love your bike. Still, you've got to be prepared, and when it comes to keeping your bike, there are two levels of preparedness: prevention and emotional readiness.

Prevention

Your bike soon will become a part of you, and when that happens, you will start to take it for granted.

Don't.

If your bike is not between your legs or secure inside your home, lock it up, and lock it well. This means none of that "Lock schlock, I'm only running into the deli for a few seconds to grab a Snapple" stuff. Don't let your thirst undermine your prudence! Haven't you ever watched a nature documentary? The lion always goes for the wildebeest at the watering hole.

SECURING THE REST OF THE STUFF

Of course the rest of the components on your bike are also technically up for grabs, but generally they're less convenient to remove, and therefore less likely to get stolen. Still, it happens, especially in high-theft cities like New York, where even handlebar and stem thefts are not uncommon.

This is especially true of racing or sport bikes, because these components are easier to remove and more attractive to thieves, whereas it's the rare thief who wants the cockpit off a Dutch bike. (If someone steals a part off your Dutch bike, just follow the clog prints.)

THE RULES OF LOCKING

1. USE A GOOD LOCK.

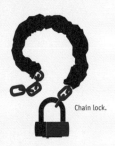

Chain lock.

Get a high-security bike lock from your local bike shop. This will likely be some sort of heavy chain, or else possibly a very stout U-lock. The advantage of a chain is that it is longer and more flexible, so you can lock your bike to a wider variety of objects, which is especially help-ful if you have a larger bike that's hard to park snugly in a bike rack. The advantage of the U-lock is that it is generally more compact and portable than a chain, and easier to mount to a bracket on your bicycle.

If you have a big bike, you probably want a chain. If you have a sporty bike, you might prefer a U-lock.

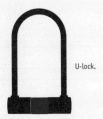

U-lock.

Do not think you can save money by making your own bike lock out of the chain and padlock you sourced from your local hardware store. This is frugal, but it is not clever. When it comes to locking your bike, frugality and security are mutually exclusive. Bike lock chains consist of links that are designed specifically to better resist bolt cutters. The chain you buy by the foot at the hardware store is not. That's why it only takes the kid selling it to you two seconds to cut it for you.

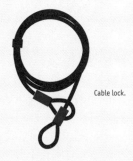

Cable lock.

Now, get a second lock for good measure.

In addition to your maximum-security lock, pick up a lighter, cheaper auxiliary lock, such as a cable lock. Use this to secure your wheel, as well as to buy a little extra time in the event a thief makes an attempt on your bike. Two locks are always better than one.

(It's also good to have a lighter lock for those trips to low-crime areas when you don't want to schlep the boat anchor with you. Just make sure it's really a low-crime area! Even the quaintest country town can be rife with thieves.)

2. LOCK THE BIKE THROUGH THE FRAME.

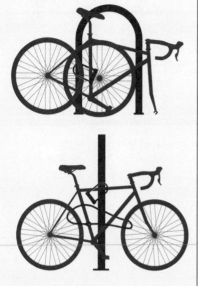

You want to be sure to pass your primary lock through your frame tubes, and not just through some easily removable part of the bike like the wheels. This way, the only way to take the bike besides opening the lock is by breaking the frame apart. If they want your bike, they're going to have to kill it first!

Also, if you can, lock one of the wheels up along with the frame. Then use that second lock for the other wheel.

3. LOCK THE BIKE *SNUGLY*.

Thieves defeat chains by cutting them, and they defeat U-locks by prying them open. You don't want to give thieves any slack, literally or figuratively. The easier it is to get a tool between the lock and your bike, the easier it is to defeat the lock.

If you're using a chain, pull it tight or wrap it around the bike multiple times before locking. If you're using a U-lock, take up as much of the inside of the U as possible by locking to something stout, putting the lock around the thickest tube on your frame, or locking your frame and your wheel at the same time.

Another good reason to lock your bike snugly is to keep it from falling over, where it might get stepped on, tripped over, or flattened by a car.

4. INSPECT THE OBJECT TO WHICH YOU'RE LOCKING.

Locking a bike isn't like locking a car, where you just push a button on a key fob and walk away. Locking a bike is a hands-on and brains-on job. It's a logic problem, a visual-spatial intelligence test. Here's what I mean: Once you've locked your bike to what appears to be a suitable pole or rack, take a closer look at it. Study it. Is there a way to remove the bike without removing the lock? Can the bike and lock be lifted up and off the pole? Is the object to which you've locked the bike open-ended somewhere you're not noticing? Did you miss your frame with your lock? (It's easy to do this when you're in a hurry, especially with a U-lock.) Is the object you're locking to weak enough to break or cut?

Look at the whole puzzle and reason it through.

Then, go one step further. Grab the pole or rack and try to rock it back and forth. You'd be surprised how often something isn't firmly anchored to the ground. All too often we take it for granted that objects are permanent parts of the cityscape. Sometimes they aren't. The city can be like Legoland. It may look solid, but you never know when you can lift a street sign right out of the sidewalk.

5. SECURE YOUR COMPONENTS.

By far the most vulnerable (and valuable) components on your bike are the wheels and the saddle (including the seat post).

• **Wheels.** Remember how you taught yourself to fix a flat? It's pretty easy to remove a wheel, isn't it? You're darn right it is! Your bike may not be stealable, but a thief will grab a wheel or two for themselves as a consolation prize.

As I mentioned earlier, ideally you should have a second lock. If you've used your primary lock to secure your frame, use this secondary lock to secure the wheels—and if you can't lock both wheels, you can always lock the rear one and take the front one inside with you.

Also, remember, it takes all of five seconds to steal a front wheel, and maybe ten seconds to steal a rear wheel, since you've got to disengage it from the drivetrain. This means the front wheel is the softest target, but keep in mind that your rear wheel is more expensive to replace.

If you've got nutted axles instead of quick releases, the wheels might take a little longer to steal, but they're still very easy to nab, so don't let your nonquick-release wheels give you a false sense of security.

(Exception to the above: If you've got a Dutch bike or something similarly utilitarian where the wheels are buried under various fenders and racks, you generally don't have to worry about locking the wheels. Not only are they time-consuming to remove, but there's not much of a black market for them.)

• **Saddle and seat post.** Remember how easy it was to raise and lower your saddle? Stealing a saddle is as easy as pulling the seat post all the way out of the seat tube. And if your saddle is fancy, it will be all the more attractive to thieves, and expensive to replace.

If you don't want to install permanent saddle theft-prevention hardware on your bike (see further on), pick up a length of braided cable with loops on either end, run it through your saddle rails, and secure the loops with your primary lock. Braided cable for bikes comes in all different lengths, and if you get a long enough piece, you can secure both your saddle and one or both of your wheels with it.

If you truly want to understand how thieves prioritize what they steal, visit New York City and study the bikes locked to poles. These living timelines will tell you everything you need to know. A well-locked bike that's been there for an hour or two should be intact. A bike that's been left overnight may be missing the saddle and the front wheel. After a week, it's down to the frame, handlebars, and drivetrain. After two weeks, the handlebars are gone too, and it's just the frame, the fork, the cranks, the chain, and the headset. At this point, even normally honest people are liable to pilfer bearings from the thing as the owner has clearly given up or moved out of town (which as far as we New Yorkers are concerned are pretty much the same thing). This is why you'll see bare frames U-locked to poles all over town.

When stationary, your bike is urban roadkill, and it will be picked clean eventually.

PROTECTING MISCELLANEOUS ACCESSORIES

Lights, saddlebag, water bottles, and anything left in your basket or panniers: All of these things are easily pilfered. It's both annoying and dangerous to have to ride home shrouded in darkness because someone nabbed your light. Take these accessories inside with you.

Also, don't lock your helmet to your bike, because a dog will pee on it. I promise. Dog owners let their precious canines pee on bikes all the time; I see it every day. In fact, I saw a dog pee on my bike while I was standing right next to it.

So don't leave the helmet on there.

Emotional Readiness

No matter how well you lock your bike, there's always the possibility that a thief might manage to steal it anyway.

No bond is unbreakable. That's just physics.

However, there is an entity that defies physics. Furthermore, once you train this entity properly, you can use it to protect yourself

Permanent theft-proofing solutions

If you ride a sporting-type bike and you regularly lock it outside for longish periods, in addition to performing the full locking regimen as outlined herein, you should also install the following permanent theft-prevention solutions on your bicycle:

- **WHEEL AXLES**
  High-end method: Replace your quick-release skewers (or axle nuts) with a theft-proof locking bolt kit. Like the wheel locks on a car, these require special keyed adapters in order to remove.
  Low-end method: Keep your quick-release skewers, but attach the levers to the frame with hose clamps.

- **SADDLE**
  High-end method: Replace your seat post clamp and your saddle clamp with a theft-proof locking bolt kit.
  Low-end method: Take an old bicycle drive chain, run it through your saddle rails and around your frame, and secure it with a chain tool.

- **STEM**
  High-end method: The bolt kit again.
  Low-end method: Stick a ball bearing inside the Allen bolt head and then seal it in there with a dollop of silicone adhesive. This will make it more difficult for a thief to get an Allen key in there.

from bike theft, and no human being on Earth can ever defeat it.

I'm talking about your mind.

Think of the Dalai Lama. The Chinese stole his home country of Tibet, but he's so blissed out that he's always smiling beatifically anyway. That's because instead of denying the inevitable, he's spent many lifetimes training to transcend the fleeting nature of matter itself.

When it comes to your bike, you have to be like the Dalai Lama. Accept that your bike is just a random grouping of matter, and that at any moment the atoms that comprise it are liable to disperse again. This doesn't obviate "prevention" as an essential component of bike ownership. In fact, it reinforces it. When you're stressed out, you make mistakes, but by coming to grips with your bike's fleeting nature and liberating yourself from your crippling attachment to it, you can operate objectively and take the necessary precautions to secure it without being misled by your clouded judgment.

Every time you walk away from your bike, you should assume it's the last time you're going to see it. Bid it farewell. Give it a hug. Take a picture. This serves three purposes:

1. When you think about your bike getting stolen, you notice things you may have missed, such as the fact that you forgot to lock it—whereas when you stop thinking about it, that's when you get lazy and it disappears.

2. If every time you leave your bike you assume it's going to

Proof of ownership

So your bike has been stolen. You've cast your eyes heavenward and excoriated the Lord for forsaking you. Your bike is gone, but that doesn't mean it can't be recovered, or that you can't at least receive some form of monetary compensation. Here are some precautions to take should you ever have to reckon with that fateful day.

• **Homeowner's or renter's insurance: have it.** Make sure your bike's on your policy.

• **Photos: keep recent ones.** If your bike vanishes, you can bring them to the local bike shops and ask if anyone's seen it. Also, if you follow any local bike people on social media, you can share the photos with them as well. As bike dorks, we can't help but scrutinize every bike we see, so you never know when one of us might recognize yours.

• **Write down your bike's serial number and keep it in a safe place.** Also, keep the receipt (if you bought the bike at a shop) and all the paperwork that came with the bike. If the police recover your bike, you may have to prove to them it's yours. Or, if you catch the thief and call the cops, he will probably claim he bought the bike from someone else—in which case the burden of proof is on you.

• **Register your bike with the local precinct.** Some police departments have programs whereby you can register your bike with them. If they do, make sure you sign up.

disappear, then you're surprised to find it still there when you return, which makes every trip you take and errand you run like getting a new bike!

3. If it does get stolen, at least you have a recent photo of your bike to show to the police.

SACRIFICIAL LAMB

Finally, if you do need to lock your bike outside regularly, the best prevention against theft is for it to be as crappy a bike as you can possibly tolerate riding. If possible, leave the crappy bike for locking up, and save your fancy bike for those recreational rides, when the bike will be spending most of its time safely beneath you. There are various formulas to determine how many bikes you should own, but the most useful one is: as many bikes as you want plus one really crappy one.

TRANSPORTING YOUR BIKE

Sooner or later you'll want to take your bike on some kind of honeymoon. How do you travel with your bike and how can you be sure to keep it safe in transit?

Besides adorning your bike with a Saint Christopher medallion, here are several ways to protect it when you're on the road.

Going by Car
ROOF RACKS

Roof racks are great. They're stable. They keep the bike out of the way and leave plenty of room inside the car for your other gear. Unfortunately, they work so well in keeping the bike out of your way that it's very easy to forget it's there until that second-too-late when you drive into a low overpass, concrete awning, or garage door, at which point your bike is reduced to a twisted wreck, often taking your rack and bits of your car along with it.

So, if you put your bike on a roof rack, do whatever you have to do to remind yourself that it's up there. Maybe this means putting a sign or a traffic cone in the driveway, or a picture of your bike on the dashboard with "Don't mangle me" written across it in big red letters.

Also, *know your clearance!* Measure the height of your car when your bike's on top of it, and keep this information somewhere in the vehicle at all times. That way, when you see a "Low Clearance" sign, you know whether or not you'll make it through without decapitating your bicycle.

Finally, *know yourself!* Are you the forgetful sort? Are you constantly losing track of your keys? Do you use Find My Phone more often than your actual phone? If so, the roof rack may not be for you. Consider other options.

HITCH RACKS/TRUNK RACKS

There are some good reasons to keep your bike behind your car instead of on top of it: less wind drag and better fuel economy, easier to remove the rack from the car when you don't need it, and virtually no chance of decapitating your bike.

Of course, this doesn't mean your bike is out of danger back there, since you can always get rear-ended. Plus, it can always fall victim to a parking mishap—if your parallel parking skills are not finely honed, that crunching sound is probably your bike.

THE IMPORTANCE OF PROPER INSTALLATION

Before mounting your bike to any sort of rack, make sure you've installed the rack properly. Then, when you put the bike on the rack, make sure you've done that properly too. If you screw any of this up, here are the three likely scenarios, from best to worst:

- Bike falls over, dents your car
- Bike flies off car, gets destroyed
- Bike flies off car on highway at high speed, terrible things happen, all because you didn't fasten your roof rack properly. Nice job.

INSIDE THE CAR

So you've got plenty of room for the bike in the car. Therefore, you've decided not to bother with a rack of any kind. Good for you! This is the safest automotive transport method for your bicycle, and as a bonus it's also the most fuel efficient.

But don't get complacent, because while your bike may be safe in the car while the car is moving, the only thing that separates it from a thief when it's parked is some auto glass. I get it. After seven hours of driving, you may not feel like removing your carefully stowed bicycle from the car when you arrive at the motel. Instead, you may decide to just leave it hidden under a blanket or something.

Don't.

Would you leave your cat, dog, or child in the car overnight? No, you wouldn't. So don't do it with your bicycle either, unless you want to find it gone the next morning.

Even if it's invisible in the trunk, it's not safe, because the places where you stop and rest on long road trips are exactly the same places thieves like to rummage through parked cars.

A note on theft

Most roof rack systems allow you to install some sort of lock cylinder. You should do this. However, that doesn't mean you should leave your bike on your rack unattended for long periods. All it takes is a screwdriver to defeat the flimsy little luggage-quality lock cylinder you'll find on most of these bike racks.

Your rack is for transporting your bike, not parking your bike.

Also, even if you don't leave your bike on the rack, keep in mind that thieves might also steal the rack itself. This is especially true of roof racks, which are prized as a fashion accessory by the sorts of people who drive tricked-out Honda Civics and Volkswagen Golfs—bike racks are basically like flat-brim baseball caps for cars. Therefore, there is a robust black market for stolen roof racks, and if you park your car outdoors, you might want to remove your roof rack when you're not using it, or else opt for some other system entirely.

Going by Plane

Here's a fact: Besides altercations with motorists, traveling by air with a bicycle is the most frustrating cycling experience you'll have.

(It's also the most frustrating air-travel experience you'll have besides traveling with a baby.)

The first thing you'll learn is that most carriers charge some kind of fee for flying with your bike, and the size of that fee can range from eyebrow raising to shocking.

The next thing you'll discover is that there's absolutely no logic behind the fee, and that they're simply applying it because "bike." It has nothing to do with fuel consumption or baggage handling or any other bogus reason they might give you when you start complaining during check-in. Even if your bicycle case is the size, weight, and shape of a typical suitcase, they will still hit you with that bike fee, because "bike."

(Of course, most airline fees seem punitive and arbitrary, but this makes the bike fee no less frustrating.)

But you're thinking, "Hey, I'm going on vacation, and I want to ride my own bike. I'll just suck it up and pay the fee." You carefully pack your bicycle in a special travel case, pay the fee, and check the case in at the airport.

What you also need to know is that if you're traveling from or to the United States, there's a little agency called the TSA. They keep us safe by checking our luggage, including your bike case, for drugs and bombs. They'll leave a little paper calling card in your bike case after they've opened it up and gone through it. That's how you know they're the ones who messed up your tidy packing job by pulling everything out and forcing it back in again like they were stuffing a turkey. This can sometimes result in damage to your components, since packing a bike is like surgery—there's only one right way to put everything back.

And what of that case? Well, generally speaking there are two kinds of bicycle travel cases: hard and soft. The hard case theoretically offers more protection for your bike, but then you've got a

Easy solutions to traveling with a bike

1. RENT OR BORROW A BIKE

Yes, if you rent or borrow you won't be riding *your* bike, but you won't have to go through all the hassle and cost of transporting your bike. Renting a bike can often be cheaper than paying the airline fees, and all you've got to bring with you are your helmet, shoes, pedals, and a few items of Lycra. Contact the bike shops at your destination and see if they rent bikes. Also, we're living in the future now, so you can always try a bike-sharing app. After all, you probably found your room on Airbnb and have an Uber waiting at the airport, so you might as well use the bicycle equivalent too while you're at it.

2. GET A TRAVEL BIKE

If you travel with your bike a lot, you should consider buying a travel bike. These are ordinary full-size bikes that feature hinges or couplers in the tubing that allow you to break down the frame and fit everything inside a case that's no larger than the typical airline maximum size limit.

Different manufacturers use different methods for building travel bikes, but a well-designed bike with couplers will perform just as well as a "regular" bike, and indeed the ride will be virtually indistinguishable, which means there's no reason you can't use this travel bike as your everyday bike as well. Furthermore, if your current nontravel bike is made of steel, you may even be able to have a professional frame builder add couplers to it so you can take it with you wherever you go.

Of course, a good travel bike (or travel bike conversion) isn't cheap, but if you fly a lot it will eventually pay for itself, and in the meantime, you'll appreciate the convenience.

big heavy case to schlep around with you, not to mention to store both at your final destination and in your home when it's not in use. The soft case is lighter, easier to maneuver in the airport, and easier to fold up and stuff in the trunk of a rental car or under the bed at home, but, well, it's soft—so it's easier for the airline to damage your precious bike.

SEMI-PRO TIPS FOR FLYING WITH BIKES

• **Dodging fees.** As I mentioned, airlines almost always charge a bike fee regardless of the size of your case, because "bike."

So, if at all possible, don't tell them it's a bike.

I'm not telling you to *lie*. I'm just saying be a bit stingy with the truth.

Of course, if you've got a giant oversized case, you're going to pay additional fees no matter what. But if you've got a travel bike in a nondescript, nonoversized case and the airline attendant wants to know what's in it, then you want to be vague. For example, I like to say it's part of a display, which implies I'm on my way to some kind of trade show.

This is not a lie, since at some point I'm going to lean the bike against something and somebody's going to look at it. That I might

also use this display for recreational purposes by sitting on top of it while it's rolling is merely circumstantial.

Also, a good way to make sure the airline doesn't ask, "What's in the case?" in the first place is to not look like a gigantic bike dork. So don't wear Oakleys and a RAGBRAI T-shirt to the airport, and cover up that bicycle tattoo while you're at it.

And what about your case? When shopping, choose a case that looks as little like sporting goods as possible. No bright colors or logos, and of course no pictures of bikes. You want something plain and black that alludes to nothing more fee-inducing than socks and underwear.

Most important, *weigh your case once it's packed*. If you're over the airline's weight allowance, all this subterfuge will be for naught.

• **Protecting your bike.** Your bike case may or may not come with some form of padding, but

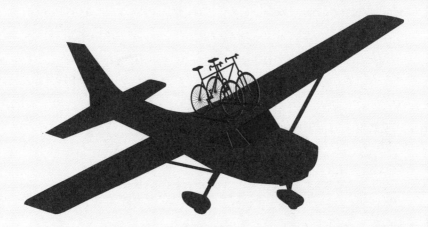

either way you should also go to the hardware store and get some foam pipe insulation. This stuff is great for protecting frame tubes, especially from cosmetic damage.

As for structural damage, your frame is at its most vulnerable when the wheels are removed, because without them the fork and chainstays can be compressed, causing them to bend or break.

New frames and bicycles are shipped with little plastic brace inserts in the fork ends and dropouts to keep this from happening. Your bike shop probably has a zillion of them lying around. Go ask for some and use them whenever you pack your bike.

• **Not putting all your eggs in one cliché.** If you're flying somewhere to ride your bike in a sporting fashion, you're going to need to bring clothes and tools and shoes and a helmet and everything else that goes with it.

It's a good idea to stick a lot of this stuff in your bike case along with your bike—assuming you can do so without exceeding the weight limit. Not only is it less to carry, but you can also use the clothing to help pad and protect the frame.

However, it's always possible your bike case will be lost or delayed, so it's never a terrible idea to keep your shoes and pedals and maybe even a pair of shorts and a jersey in your carry-on. That way, if you're forced to borrow someone else's bike, at least you won't have to borrow their shorts and shoes too.

• **Packing your tools.** You had to take your bike apart in order to pack it, so of course you've packed all the tools you need in order to put it back together again, right?

Of course you did.

You're not going to be running around a hotel at 3:00 AM looking for a pedal wrench, right? You're smarter than that.

Also, after you arrive at your destination and assemble your bike, it will almost certainly require some additional adjustment. Therefore, in addition to the usual Allen keys, you should also bring a spoke wrench, because wheels often get knocked out of true while in transit.

You should also be sure to bring a pump, but keep in mind that despite what people may say on the Internet you do *not* have to deflate your tires before flying. They will *not* explode. In fact, you should top them off before you leave so you don't have to deal with it when you get where you're going. The only reason to deflate your tires before flying is if your wheels will not fit in the case otherwise, which can often happen with smaller travel bike cases.

Another option is no case at all. Some traveling cyclists use a cardboard bike box (your bike shop will be happy to give you one if you ask nicely), and still others will simply wrap their naked bikes in plastic. Anecdotally, baggage handlers are more careful with these bikes because they see it's in fact a bike and not just a bunch of underwear. This may or may not be true. It's also obviously a lot cheaper than using a case, which is good, since you'll need the savings to offset all those exorbitant bike fees. Still, you've got to pack the bike carefully, and you're always gambling on what the bike is going to look like when you meet it on the other side.

On top of all this, regardless of your packing method, you need to pay close attention to your itinerary and even the size of the aircraft. If one of the legs of the flight involves a small plane, there may not be room on it for your bike, in which case the airline may decide to send it along later—which can seriously screw up your carefully planned cycling vacation.

Going by Train

When it comes to cycling day trips, no two forms of transportation complement each other quite as nicely as bikes and trains. Sure, it's easy to throw your bike in the car, but there's always a certain amount of shame involved in driving to the ride. There's nothing wrong with it per se, but it can feel like sort of a cop-out, like visiting a foreign city and only eating at Subway.

The train, on the other hand, is romantic. You roll your bike on board, the rhythm of the rails lulls you as you escape the city's orbit, and then you roll right off and into the countryside. All that's missing is the tweed.

Unfortunately, rail travel isn't quite what it used to be—especially if you live in the United States, where after World War II we basically said screw trains and focused all our infrastructure efforts on cars.

The upshot of this is that trains often lack amenities for cyclists.

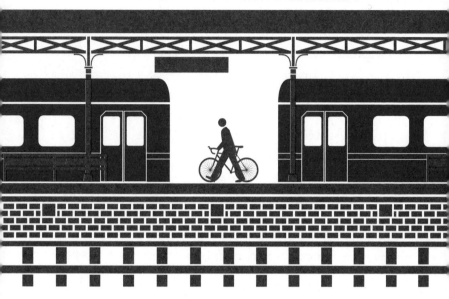

Therefore, it's crucial to check with your railroad beforehand and find out what rules they have for traveling with bikes. Sometimes you can take bikes on some trains but not on others. Sometimes you can take bikes on some train *cars* but not on others. Sometimes you need a special reservation. Sometimes you need a permit. Sometimes you can't take bikes on trains at all. So make sure you research every leg of your trip, because you don't want to board a train home only to be refused by a conductor.

As for local trains, such as subways, these can be quite handy in

A warning about gatherings

Take extra care when traveling to big cycling events. You are part of a herd now. This makes you extra vulnerable. Thieves love herds, because not only are there lots of bikes, but the first thing you do when you join a herd is switch off your brain. So don't leave your bike on or in your car. Don't leave it sitting out on your host's porch. Don't leave it in the lobby or hallway of the hotel. Pay attention at the rest area or at the coffee shop. Bring a lock with you and use it. The only thing you lose at a bike event should be your dignity.

a pinch—like, say, the skies have opened up and you don't feel like riding home. So make a point of knowing the bike rules where you live. Also, be considerate. For example, in New York City you're technically allowed to take your bike onto the subway at all times, but in practice, if you attempt to do this during rush hour you're a serious jerk.

Going by Bus

Depending on your municipality, your local bus may be equipped with bicycle racks. If so, lucky you.

If, however, you're going on a long interstate bus trip, I can only assume you're either touring with a rock band or you've hit rock bottom and are escaping à la Ratso Rizzo, in which case you almost certainly sold your bike off years ago.

In either case you're on your own.

Chapter 4

OPERATING YOUR BIKE

The bicycle is one of the most useful, powerful, unregulated vehicles you can buy.

You may have noticed when purchasing your bike that nobody asked you for your license or registration or insurance certificate or even whether or not you knew how to ride the thing. You don't need special training or permission to purchase and ride a bicycle, which is good. However, not everyone who purchases a bike, and this may include you, has much experience riding a bike, which is not so good.

Because in many places, cycling is a marginalized form of transportation. A lot of us learn to ride as a child and then abandon the bike for a car as soon as we're old enough to drive. When you finally return to the bike as an adult, you're still effectively that ten-year-old pedaling around in the cul-de-sac. The result is that too many cyclists fail to comport themselves in a safe and mature fashion, which is another way of saying that they're crappy riders.

Bad habits need to be corrected quickly with new knowledge and experience. To a large extent, the bicycle itself is going to be your best instructor. Cars are poor instructors. They are soft, mushy, and climate controlled, which promotes mental and physical laziness. Sure, you have to earn a license to drive one, but that's a pretty low bar considering you only have to pass a driver's test once in your lifetime and it's only slightly harder than aligning your window with the loudspeaker at the drive-thru. Bicycles, on the other hand, leave you exposed to the elements and respond to even the tiniest bit of operator feedback, so they work well only when you're fit and alert. It doesn't take long to figure out what you're doing wrong. If you screw up the clothing part, you get cold. If you screw up the riding part, you fall down. You're tested and retested on the bike every day, and proficiency comes in relatively short order.

Still, there are a lot of potential mistakes you can work to avoid, so it pays to familiarize yourself with the basics of bicycle operation.

HOW A BICYCLE WORKS

Here are all the ways you can make your bike move.

MOVING THE BICYCLE FORWARD

Situate the bicycle between your legs. Next, rotate cranks with one foot until one pedal is slightly in front of the bottom bracket. Position the ball of your foot over the pedal spindle and push. This will get the bike rolling. Once you've got sufficient momentum to keep the bike moving without falling over, position your other foot identically and send power to your bicycle's drivetrain as desired by pressing on each pedal in a rhythmic alternating fashion.

This is called "pedaling."

Pedal using the ball of your foot. Don't pedal with the arch or heel of your foot; that's for beachcombers and freelance recycling collectors.

MOVING THE BICYCLE BACKWARD

Unless you're thinking of taking up artistic cycling, or perhaps bike polo, there is no reason you would ever need to ride a bicycle backward, so don't worry about it.

WATCHING WHERE YOU'RE GOING

While you're riding, you should always be scanning for obstacles.

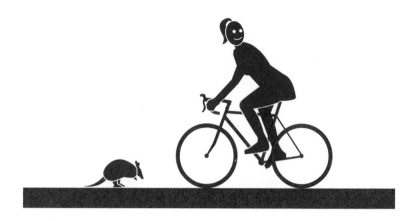

Think of yourself as a submarine in hostile waters, constantly sending out sonar pulses. Motorcycle instructors use the acronym SEE—search, evaluate, and execute—and this applies to us cyclists as well. Not only do you need to be aware of what's going on up the road, but you also need to be aware of the road surface immediately ahead of your front tire. You're looking for potholes, road seams, armadillos—anything that's liable to take you down.

The bicycle does not allow your attention to wander, and a momentary lapse is all it takes to hit a pedestrian or plow into a car door.

CHANGING DIRECTION

You might hear people say, "The bicycle goes where you look." This is true. It's why the Tour de France peloton looks so graceful from above—each rider is fixed on the haunches of the rider ahead, so they all move as though they are one. If you're busy admiring your own reflection in a shop window instead of looking at the road ahead, you'll drift over toward the curb and run into the rear of a parked car. How do you look now?

You'll also hear people talk about "countersteering," which they'll explain by saying something like "Push left to go right." If that sounds vexingly Mr. Miyagi-ish to you, don't worry about it. It only means you need to sort of lean into the turns, and that if you wrench the handlebars like you're playing a video game or using a post hole auger, you're going to fall down.

When steering, you want to grip the bars, but not squeeze them. A death grip on the bars causes stiffness in your arms. You need those arms to be loose so they can help absorb shock and bumps from the road. But if your grip is too loose, hitting a big bump will cause you to lose your grip altogether, which could end with you on the ground.

A lot of people don't realize that steering a bike also comes from using your thighs, so you'll want to develop some groinal dexterity. Think of your saddle as a rudder that you steer with your undercarriage. To get a sense of how this works, push your bike along the sidewalk with just one hand on the saddle. Notice how you can use the input from your hand to control the bike. This groinal dexterity is also what will allow you to master no-handed riding.

SLOWING AND STOPPING

Your bicycle should be equipped with front and rear brakes. If it isn't, take it back. Most of the stopping power is in your front brake, so that one's the most important, though it's good practice to use both.

Keep in mind that suddenly applying the front brake can send you flying over the bars. Particularly when braking on steep descents, it's best to keep steady pressure on your front brake and fine-tune your speed with your rear brake.

Like many cars, your bicycle is equipped with an antilock braking system (ABS), but unlike your car, that system is your brain. If you sense your wheels locking up and losing traction, ease up on the levers slightly and then reapply the brake gradually. If you feel your rear wheel lifting, ease up on the front and apply the rear. If you feel your rear wheel skidding, ease up on the rear and apply the front.

No matter what kind of brakes you have, they use friction to

A note on hand signaling

There's a whole crazy elaborate system of "official" hand signals you're supposed to use when riding a bike. Don't bother to learn these. Nobody understands them. What *is* important to learn is that if you're riding in traffic you need to signal your turns. To do this, point clearly and obviously in the direction you intend to go.

The purpose of signaling is to mitigate ambiguity to the greatest extent possible. Everybody understands pointing.

Using archaic cycling hand signals is like speaking in Elizabethan English—technically correct, but entirely bewildering.

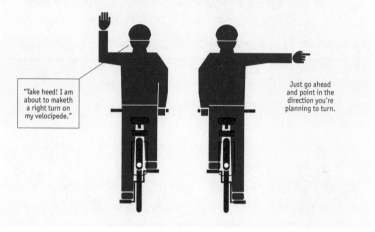

"Take heed! I am about to maketh a right turn on my velocipede."

Just go ahead and point in the direction you're planning to turn.

stop your bike, and the result of that friction is heat, which can cause your braking power to fade. So if you're descending for a really long time, it's a good idea to vary your braking pressure to allow the braking surface to cool. Braking on long descents should involve both hands in a constant state of firm yet gentle modulation—you should be working the levers like Patrick Swayze in the pottery wheel scene in *Ghost*.

If you're riding a bicycle with drop bars, you'll get far more stopping power by braking from the drops.

Take the time to familiarize yourself with your bicycle's brakes. Ride up and down the block. Try the front. Try the rear. Practice stopping short. Skid. See what it takes to lock them up. See what it feels like when your rear wheel comes off the ground. If there's too much lever travel before the brakes engage, then adjust your brakes accordingly. Rush-hour traffic is not a good place to learn the nuances of your braking system. Get to know it before you head out into the real world.

ATTIRE AND EQUIPMENT

Before we talk about proper attire, let's have "the helmet talk," because lots of people are going to tell you that you need to wear one or else you will die.

These people are wrong.

Not that you won't die, it's just that death doesn't really care what you're wearing on your head.

Helmets

No subject pits cyclist against cyclist or sets the cycling blogosphere ablaze more than bicycle helmets. Some cyclists insist that straddling a bicycle without first strapping on a helmet is an act of foolhardiness akin to letting an unsupervised toddler cook scrambled eggs. Others believe that helmets are mostly ineffectual, and that forcing cyclists to wear foam caps is a cop-out that excuses reckless drivers and distracts from the need for street redesigns.

The truth is that helmets are not as effective in preventing head injuries as we've been led to believe. Here in the United States, for example, both the Centers for Disease Control and Prevention and the National Highway Traffic Safety Administration used to cite a study claiming that bicycle helmets reduce your risk of head injury by eighty-five percent. It turns out that this study is seriously biased and badly flawed, and after being petitioned by the Washington Area Bicyclists Association, both agencies are now withdrawing the claim under the federal Data Quality Act.

Other studies indicate bicycle helmets yield results way below the eighty-five percent figure, and some researchers and cycling advocates claim they're hardly effective at all. People often cite a split or cracked helmet as evidence that it saved them from brain injury in a crash. "See? That would have been my skull!" However, cracking can be a sign that the helmet did *not* do its job. Helmets are made of foam, and that foam has to compress in order to slow the linear acceleration of the brain. If the helmet cracks, the foam did not compress, and if the foam did not compress, it didn't do anything for your brain.

Furthermore, sometimes helmets crack from some glancing, angular impact that might not have caused any injury at all—and

|||||||||||||||||||||||

STYLES OF HELMETS

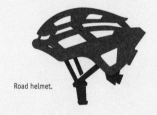

Road helmet.

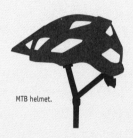

MTB helmet.

• ROAD RACING

These are generally very light with lots of vents, though recently "aero" has become fashionable with the roadies so the vents are disappearing again. (It used to be you paid a premium for vents; now you pay a premium for no vents. Go figure.) Either way, racing helmets are light and comfortable, though they can be expensive, and if you're commuting you may feel a bit strange wearing one with a blazer.

• MOUNTAIN BIKE

Depending on what sort of mountain biking you're doing, this can be anything from a road racing helmet with a visor (mountain bikers often favor visors so they don't get slapped in the face by tree branches) to a full-face affair virtually indistinguishable from a motocross helmet. Unless you're downhilling or launching yourself off massive dirt jumps, a road helmet and a mountain bike helmet are pretty much interchangeable.

• URBAN

Various companies offer stylish helmets for city riding—or at least stylish by safety gear standards. Usually they look like batting helmets, or skateboard helmets, or something a European police officer might wear. In any case, if you're concerned

in fact sometimes you hit your head in a crash *because* you're wearing a helmet. To understand how that happens, next time you get dressed for a ride, put your helmet on first. I guarantee you'll bump your helmeted head at least three times while you're putting on the rest of your gear, because your foam-encased head is now significantly larger.

Still, at some point you'll be talking to someone who will tell you that you're an idiot for not wearing a helmet, such as a doctor or a nurse. "I work in the ER. I see brain injuries all the time!" This is compelling, but keep in mind they only see the injured riders,

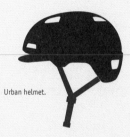

Urban helmet.

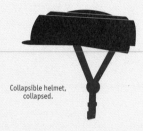

Collapsible helmet, collapsed.

about aesthetics, these types of safety hats will go better with your city or commuting bike and street attire than a racing helmet.

• **COLLAPSIBLE**
Helmets can be a bit unwieldy to carry around, which is why people often leave them on their bikes when they park—or else on their

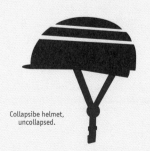

Collapsibe helmet, uncollapsed.

heads, which makes them look extremely cautious while they're browsing the supermarket. Collapsible helmets attempt to address the portability problem by reducing the bulk by a few inches, so maybe you can at least fit the damn thing in your bag.

• **HELMETS THAT LOOK LIKE HATS**
Yes, at least one company offers covers that disguise your helmet as a hat. If you want to wear, say, a preternaturally stiff-looking tweed cap with an inexplicable chinstrap that looks at least four sizes too big for you, then go right ahead. But just be aware that you're not fooling anybody. They're like the hair plugs of bicycle safety gear.

not the ones who walk away. Furthermore, medical doctors are not physicists. They don't always know the particulars of how the crash occurred or the forces that were at work.

But it's not just about safety. Excessive faith in helmets has also resulted in an outsourcing of responsibility on the part of both drivers and cyclists: Drivers get to blame their victims, and cyclists are duped into thinking their responsibilities begin and end with strapping a foam buoy to their heads. Worst of all, it can lead to mandatory helmet laws, which do little for rider safety but do a lot to discourage cycling. (When Australia implemented a mandatory helmet law in the 1990s, cycling trips dipped by thirty to forty percent.)

So all this means you shouldn't wear a helmet, right?

Not at all!

Rather, it means you might want to abandon the notion that wearing a helmet automatically equals "responsible cyclist." Think of the helmet less as the difference between life and death and more as a ceremonial headdress that helps you prepare mentally for your ride. For example, if you're putting on special shoes and special shorts and a special jersey with little pockets in the back and you plan to spend hours on end riding at various speeds, by all means don your plastic speed hat too. If nothing else, it helps put you in the right frame of mind and reminds you that high-speed cycling can be particularly dangerous if you're not safety-minded.

However, if you're just hopping on the bike in your street clothes to ride around town, you might as well leave it at home, just as long as you plan to ride smart—because while a helmet might remind you to be safe, it might also give you a false sense of security. Furthermore, studies have shown that your helmet may also give *drivers* a false sense of security, in that they will pass you more closely.

After all, you're wearing a helmet, and helmets are "eighty-five percent effective," so if they crash into you they won't hurt you, right?

And of course, if you're doing some crazy downhill mountain

biking you should certainly wear a helmet, and probably a full-face one at that, because riding into a tree is riding into a tree, so you might as well have something between the bark and your face. "Regular" mountain biking also warrants a helmet, since you're almost guaranteed to fall down at low speed at least once per ride, and these sorts of low-speed spills are the situations in which bicycle helmets are most effective. Plus, most parks with mountain bike trails require helmets, and you don't want to run afoul of the land managers who decide our trail access.

Most important, if you do wear a helmet, *wear it properly*. Visit the bike path on a typical day and you'll notice at least half the people on it have their helmets on wrong—either the straps are way too loose, the helmet's riding way back on the head like a cowboy's hat on a hot day, or else the thing's just plain backward. Not only is an improperly worn helmet ineffective, but it can actually be *more dangerous*, since if it's too loose it can choke you in a crash. Seriously.

So wear your helmet right or don't wear it at all.

Practical Riding

Every year around Bike Month (May) the newspapers and magazines run lists of "essential" bike commuting gear that, were you to purchase it all, would run into the thousands of dollars.

Please.

If your commute is short—let's say under a half hour—don't even think about special commuting attire. Just wear the same stuff you would if you were walking to work. If your bike doesn't have a chainguard, then roll up your pants. If you don't want to wrinkle your pants because they're slacks, then spend a few bucks on a pant cuff retainer. Also, you might need a new bag if you have to carry a lot of stuff with you. That's really it.

If, however, you're commuting closer to an hour or more each way, then you're putting in some real saddle time. This will take its toll on your appearance. Wheel splatter, wrinkled clothing, sweat stains . . . If you're not careful you might arrive at the office looking like someone chased you there.

FENDERS

The first line of defense against filth is your bike. If at all possible install full fenders, both front and rear. Even if it rains while you're riding, they'll save you from the worst of it, because the water that falls from the sky is much cleaner than the water that flies back up from the street and onto your rear.

SADDLE

Speaking of the seat of your pants, mile after mile of cycling will take its toll, so pay attention to your saddle. Embroidered or textured seat covers will wear through pants fabric more quickly than smooth ones, and if you wear jeans you'll eventually be walking around with the ghost image of a saddle on your posterior. Smooth plastic saddles free from embroidery will be the most gentle on your pants. Smooth leather saddles are exceedingly comfortable, but when they get wet they can cause embarrassing discoloration that makes it look like you sat in minestrone soup (or worse) so take care to make sure yours stays dry. Cover your saddle when your bike is parked outside. Various companies will sell you pants with reinforced crotches specifically for cycling, but they're often expensive and no garment lasts forever, so if they're beyond your budget don't worry about it. The inexpensive jeans with a bit of stretch in them that they sell at certain young-skewing casual-wear chain stores happen to work very well for commuting.

STAYING WARM

There are two key ways to stay warm on the bike: blocking the wind and staying dry. You want a wind- and water-resistant outer layer, an insulated middle later, and a light base layer to draw the sweat away from your skin. None of this stuff needs to be bicycle-specific. A Windbreaker or rain jacket, a wool sweater, and a light undershirt or thermal will keep you warm even in freezing temperatures.

You'll want a jacket with a high collar to protect your neck. Neck gaiters can come in handy when it's very cold, or you can just wear a scarf, which has the added benefit of further insulating your chest. You can also use these to cover your face if it's particularly blustery outside.

Your delicate Palmolive-soaked hands are just sitting out there in the wind like two tropical birds on a perch, so always carry insulated gloves—or better yet, mittens, since they're much warmer and you don't need great manual dexterity to operate a bicycle anyway. A hat is also essential, and wool generally works best. Make sure the hat can cover your ears, because frozen ears will ruin your ride. If you wear a helmet, it shouldn't be too hard to find a hat that will fit underneath it—and for extra protection put some clear packing tape over the helmet vents. That way you'll get a whole greenhouse effect going on around your head.

Your toes are also very vulnerable to the cold, because like your fingers they're mostly just sitting there doing nothing. Leave the breathable mesh at home. Boots and wool socks should be sufficient in all but the coldest temperatures. Foot retention systems such as clipless pedals or toe clips and straps are not ideal for commuting because they limit your footwear choices—and anyway you're riding to work, not climbing Alpe d'Huez. (Unless of course you work on top of Alpe d'Huez.)

STAYING COOL

Dressing to stay cool isn't very complicated—all you have to do is wear the least amount of clothing you can get away with without being fired or arrested. Additionally, scope out a shady route to work if possible, as this can make a tremendous difference on your comfort level. If you can avoid hills, that's even better. Leave early—not only is it cooler, but you can ride slower. Rushing leads to overheating, and if you time trial it to work, you'll spend that first hour at your desk sweating.

Speaking of sweating, always keep an extra shirt either in your bag or at work in case you sweat through yours on the way.

Most important, *get that bag off your back*! Install some kind of rack on your bike instead. Move the load from your body to the bicycle.

CLOTHING FIT

When you start commuting on a sporting-type bicycle you'll learn that clothing fits differently when you're on the bike. Sleeves ride up your arms. Jackets ride up your back. Pant waists work their way down, and you show everybody your coin slot.

Make sure your jacket accommodates a riding position. Choose shirts that will cover your lower back when you're leaning forward a bit. Wear a belt. Opt for pants that have a bit of stretch in them—I'm not saying wear yoga pants, but you want something that's going to give you the freedom and mobility to spin your legs comfortably for a while.

If you don't want to deal with any of that, then opt for a bicycle that puts you in an upright position, such as a Dutch bike. You may also be able to swap the handlebars on your sporty-type bike to put you in a more upright riding position.

SKIRTS AND STEP-THROUGHS

"I like to wear skirts. What should I do?"

If you want to commute in a skirt—or you just value comfort, practicality, and ease of use—you should seriously consider a step-through bicycle, or what in the old days people used to call a "girl's bike." The chief advantage of the step-through is that instead of swinging your leg over the bike like you're doing the cancan, you just step right through the frame as the name suggests. Not only is this much easier, but you don't have to show the world your underwear.

Another great thing about a step-through bike is that it's far easier to mount and dismount when the bike is loaded (even the

STUFF YOU DON'T NEED AND STUFF YOU MIGHT WANT

• STUFF YOU DON'T NEED

—Special bike-specific jackets with weird bike lock key pockets on the wrist and internal routing for your headphone cable

You will never use any of that stuff, I promise.

—Clipless-compatible shoes disguised as casual wear

Come on. Just use flat pedals.

—Handlebar-mounted smart-phone brackets

Seriously, you don't have to use your phone every second of the day. One of the best things about cycling is that it offers a respite from constant connectivity. If you need to use the phone, just stop for a few minutes.

• STUFF YOU MIGHT WANT

—A rearview mirror

Some mount to your helmet, others mount to your handlebars. They are considered dorky by some, but who cares? There's nothing wrong with knowing what's behind you.

—A kickstand or centerstand

Another accessory too often dismissed as "dorky," a kickstand or centerstand can be extremely handy for the practical cyclist. They have no place on racing bikes, but if you use your bike for riding around town, why search for a wall or a rack every time you want to get off your bike? Centerstands are especially useful when you carry a lot of stuff, because they allow you to load the bike without it falling over.

—A video camera

More and more companies are making video cameras that mount to your bicycle. Many cyclists use them to make tedious movies of their mountain biking sessions that they then upload to YouTube, but their most important function is as potential evidence if you're wronged by a motorist or officer of the law. Granted, even video evidence isn't always enough to get someone in trouble, but at the very least you can shame them in public, which can be just as vindicating.

most experienced cyclist has dumped a bike with a full basket or panniers), and you can also easily stop and straddle the bike in order to make adjustments to whatever load you're carrying, or to take a phone call as the case may be.

Additionally, you should make sure your step-through is equipped with skirt guards, which are a common feature on Dutch-style bikes. These are essentially plastic covers on either side of the rear wheel that keep your voluminous gown, long coat, or prehensile tail from getting caught in the spokes. Otherwise your skirt could fly off like in some dirty old-timey Mutoscope.

Fun Riding

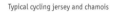

If you're riding for fun, you should wear whatever you are comfortable in and whatever makes you happy, be it a skinsuit or a chicken suit.

However, the sooner you come to terms with wearing Lycra the better.

You may think stretchy bike clothes look silly (because they kind of do), but really, if you're spending hours on the bike there's nothing better. It's light. It's comfortable. It dries in seconds.

Typical cycling jersey and chamois

Another benefit to Lycra is that it's modular, and you can wear it all year round.

Lycra clothing can be expensive, but you really only need a few pieces, and because you only wear it on the bike (or at least most people do, but if you want to wear cycling shorts on the subway that's totally up to you) it will last you a long time just as long as you don't crash. To maximize the life of your expensive bike clothes, don't put them in the dryer—which there's not much reason to do anyway since it dries so quickly.

Here's how it works, from hot to cold:

1. Shorts and jersey
2. Knee warmers and arm warmers
3. Leg warmers and vest
4. Tights, jacket, shoe covers, gloves

When you're hot, you just remove pieces of clothing and stuff them in your jersey pockets, and when you're cold, you put them right back on again.

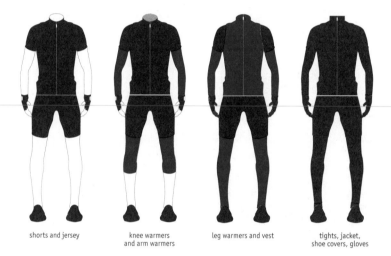

shorts and jersey

knee warmers and arm warmers

leg warmers and vest

tights, jacket, shoe covers, gloves

Despite its association with roadies, Lycra is also perfectly at home on the mountain bike trails, and while the full-face helmet set prefers to wear baggy shorts and jerseys, most go-fast cyclists wear more or less the same stuff on the trails as they do on the road.

BIB SHORTS VS. HALF SHORTS

Bib shorts have integrated suspenders, whereas half shorts do not. Bib shorts fit better and don't ride down, though they do make it more inconvenient to go to the bathroom—depending on your anatomy and which number you have to go (that's #1 or #2) you may have to partially disrobe first. Virtually all high-end shorts are going to be of the bib variety.

EYEWEAR

In the cycling industry they call this stuff "optics," by which they mean "sunglasses." Besides mitigating sun glare, eyewear also prevents all kinds of foreign objects from flying into your eyes while you ride, and it can be disconcerting to try to blink a gnat out while riding downhill at thirty-five miles per hour. You can spend huge amounts of money on cycling eyewear and lenses with tints for every conceivable lighting condition, but really any sport-oriented pair of sunglasses will work fine on bright days. If you ride in low-light situations, you can also save a lot of money by getting amber safety glasses instead of the bike-specific ones.

CYCLING CAPS

There's lots of gimmickry in cycling, but some things just work, and one of them is the cycling cap. It's timeless, and it fits under your helmet. The short, low brim won't catch the wind, but it's just enough to deflect the sun or protect your eyes from wind, rain, debris—or even the occasional tree branch if you're venturing off-road. You might even find that with a cycling cap on, you can dispense with eyewear altogether. They're also useful for hiding your helmet hair at the café.

HOW TO RIDE YOUR BIKE

Now that you're properly attired and know how to steer and use your brakes, let's get into the specifics of operating your bike under various conditions.

Commuting

Commuting is the act of regularly riding a bike to a place you wouldn't visit if you didn't have to, such as school or work. The advantages of commuting by bike are as follows:

- It's cheap.
- It keeps you healthy and fit.

- It helps relieve stress.
- You can avoid getting caught in traffic.
- You're less likely to be stuck sitting next to an exhibitionist than you are on public transportation, unless you share a tandem bicycle with an exhibitionist.

ROUTE SELECTION

Once you've decided to try commuting, the first thing to do is figure out your route. If you've been commuting by car, you already know how to get to work, but the best routes for driving are often the worst routes for cycling. If your city or town has a bike advocacy group, check out their bike map. Google's cycling directions are also fairly reliable.

Ride the route on a weekend or day off. This way you'll get a sense of how long the ride will take and you won't find yourself in a rush on a workday. Also, things like potholes, construction zones, or traffic pattern changes aren't apparent from maps, so you'll want to be able to account for them ahead of time.

Target the most pleasant route and not necessarily the fastest one.

THINGS TO LOOK FOR ON THE ROUTE:
- Bike lanes
- Tree-lined streets (for shade)
- Cafés, bars with happy hours

THINGS TO AVOID ON THE ROUTE:
- Truck routes
- Busy shopping centers
- Schools (there is no more self-absorbed driver than a parent dropping off or picking up a child)

PARKING

Unless you're riding a folding bike (which you can stick right under your desk, smiling smugly to yourself all the while) you're going

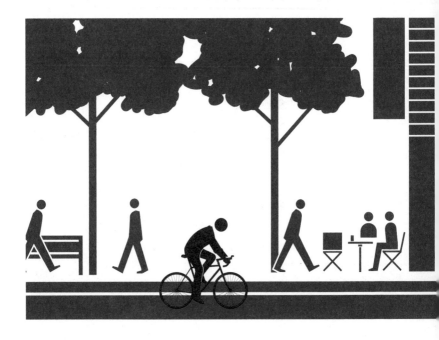

to need a place to park your bike once you arrive at your destination. You should get that all figured out before you roll up in front of your building at 9:02 AM, sweaty, late, and with no place to ditch your bike.

If your workplace has a bike room, then good for you, you're all set. If it doesn't, you may be able to bring the bike in anyway. For example, in New York City there's a law that says bikes must be allowed inside buildings of a certain size and with freight elevators. If you work in a small building or for a small company, explain to your boss that bicycle commuters like you save companies money and boost productivity because they take fewer sick days and are generally healthier, and therefore you should be allowed to keep your bike in the mailroom. (Unfortunately, you may have to live up to that promise, so if you're lazy or like to play hooky once in a while it may not be worth it.)

If you absolutely can't bring your bike inside because you work in a lousy building or for a lousy boss, then you may be able to find alternative indoor parking nearby. Some bike shops offer it,

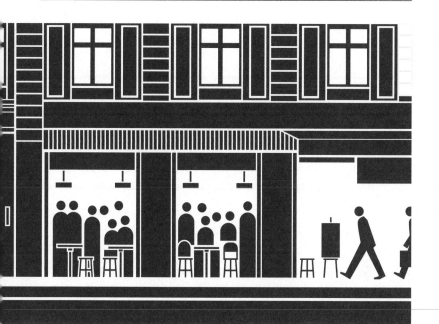

as does some of the new breed of bicycle café. You can even pay to park your bike in a garage, though that feels kind of wrong, like paying for Wi-Fi at the airport.

Then there's the street. It's free, but it comes with the obvious set of risks (see Chapter 3). Check out the bike racks around your office. Look at where others are parking. Better yet, talk to your fellow commuters. They may have some useful advice. "Lock up in front of the lobby, there's a security camera." "Don't use the pole in front of that fancy condo, the superintendent cuts the locks." "Not many people know this, but there's a bike rack inside near the loading dock." And so forth.

FRESHENING UP

Arrive at work with sufficient time to cool down or thaw out, depending on the season. If your job requires a lot of speaking, it can be difficult to do this with a frozen mouth. You don't want to blow "the big deal" because you sound like someone shot you up with Novocain and nobody can understand you. (Yes, I only know about business deals from movies and sitcoms.)

Also, bike commuting is like eating ribs: It can get a little messy, so always keep some wet wipes and a clean change of clothes handy.

COMMUTING ETIQUETTE

Riding a bicycle is exhilarating, and like any form of intoxication, this heightened sense of well-being can turn you into a jerk. And if you pair this exhilaration with the notion that you're saving the world by using an eco-friendly mode of transportation, then you can become downright insufferable as well. Therefore, it's important to remain humble and considerate, and to remember you're no better than every other person out there trying to get someplace.

Do not attempt to race or draft off of your fellow bike commuters. It's like ogling people on the subway—you think you're being discreet about it, but everyone knows you're doing it, and you come off as a creep. Plus, sitting on someone's wheel is a great way to crash into them if they have to stop. If someone attempts to

Bike commuting is not an all-or-nothing proposition

Commuting by bike may become a part of your identity, but you don't have to do it every day. It's perfectly fine to skip the bike if the weather's lousy or you just don't feel like riding that day. Nobody's judging you. Well, that's not entirely true, because the smuggest bike commuters are probably judging you, but what do you care what a bunch of quinoa eaters think?

Try to remember that *multimodalism is good.* Being a bike commuter doesn't have to mean riding exclusively from door to door. Depending on where you live and where you work, it might make more sense to integrate the bike with other forms of transit. For example, instead of riding twenty miles to work, you can ride two miles to the station and take the train the rest of the way. If there's no public transit where you live (let's hear it for the USA!) then you can even drive and ride, because there's no law that says you can't combine driving with cycling.

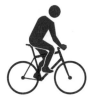
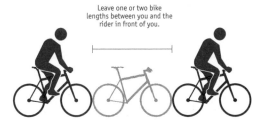

Leave one or two bike lengths between you and the rider in front of you.

race you, let them go and laugh at how silly they look as they spin away frantically.

Do not push ahead to line up in front of other cyclists at red lights. Instead, take your place at the back of the line. The rules of society do not reverse themselves just because you're on a bicycle.

KNOW YOUR RIGHTS AND RESPONSIBILITIES

Different cities and towns have different laws when it comes to bikes. For example, in Idaho they have something called the "Idaho stop." No, this is not a euphemism for a form of police brutality involving a potato. Idaho stop is the name of a law that lets cyclists treat stop signs as yield signs and red lights as stop signs. If you live in Idaho, that's the kind of thing you should know.

Not all regional bike laws are good, either. In many towns it's illegal for cyclists to ride two abreast. (How dare you be almost as wide as a car!) Seattle has a helmet law. (Yet marijuana is legal, go figure.) And in Portland, Oregon, it's illegal to ride a bike that hasn't been hand built by a bearded craftsman. (Well, that's not true, but it might as well be.)

Then there are the laws pertaining to your bike. Lights are pretty much universally mandatory. The same goes for brakes. Often you're even required to have a bell. Then there's the stuff that would probably never even occur to you, like laws that say you have to ride with at least one hand on the bars at all times. (This is the case in New York City.) Not that you shouldn't ride no-handed (it's an essential cycling skill, after all), but you should at least know all the excuses your local police have at their disposal for stopping you.

It's also important to stay connected and informed. You don't need to get involved in local bike advocacy, but you should at least follow some people who are.

See, when you drive, you take for granted that the mainstream media is going to provide you with important information: traffic reports, road closures, weather conditions, that sort of thing. It doesn't work that way with bikes. Cyclists are still marginalized in most communities, so any information you get is going to have to come from the grassroots level. This means checking in on the blogs, Facebook pages, and Twitter feeds of your local advocates and cycling clubs. You don't want to find out when you're already running late that the bike path on the bridge is closed for two weeks, or that it's covered with a sheet of ice because the local department of transportation hasn't gotten around to salting it. Fortunately, bike people love to complain, so if you follow the right ones you'll see plenty of indignant tweets about any major or minor situations before leaving the house.

Road Riding

Road riding is the act of riding a bicycle, usually one with drop bars, on public roadways for no ostensible purpose beyond recreation.

You may notice when venturing out on a road ride that many of your fellow cyclists look perturbed, consternated, or even downright miserable, which would appear to go against the very concept of recreation.

This is normal, and merely a side effect of goal-oriented recreation. The typical road cyclist is attempting to process two or three digital data streams while in a state of extreme physical exertion, and is also focusing intently on getting home to the family by a certain time "or else."

PREPARATION

When undertaking your first road ride, plan your route before heading out. Ideally, this route should incorporate a stop for food and rest at the turnaround point. You want to avoid densely populated areas and seek quiet back roads to the greatest extent possible. Motor vehicle traffic is not conducive to road cycling enjoyment. Those "Share the Road" signs may seem encouraging, but keep in mind that if the drivers were actually sharing the road, then the signs wouldn't be there in the first place.

If you live in an area where there are a sizable number of road riders, there is probably a quaint town with a café in it that serves as the default roadie destination. Heading in that direction is a good place to start, because not only is the route well established, but it will also afford you the opportunity to study the behavior of other roadies, for better or worse.

Know the climate and check the weather conditions. Just because the sky's clear doesn't mean it's going to stay that way. If you're heading out early, be aware that it might be a lot warmer in a few hours. If you'll be climbing long hills, keep in mind it might be a lot colder at the top. Dress accordingly.

The savviest road riders roll out as early as possible, both to maximize riding time and to beat the traffic. Midday road rides can be annoying because the roads are busier.

Your body will give you little warning before dehydration and glycogen depletion (colloquially known as "bonking") kick in, so plan accordingly. The key is to prepare for a big ride the day before by getting plenty to eat and drinking lots of water. Hydration is especially important. If your urine is not perfectly clear before you go to bed, then you have not drunk enough, because you cannot sufficiently rehydrate on the bike. Eat a substantial breakfast and carry both food and water with you, which you should eat and drink at regular intervals rather than waiting for your body to ask for it, because by then it's often too late.

You can buy all sorts of energy bars and gels and boutique

waffle snacks and powdered drinks if you'd like, but that stuff's expensive and gimmicky, and for most rides it's hard to beat water, bananas, nuts, granola, fig bars, dried fruit, and all that other stuff that has been sustaining humans for centuries and millennia.

If you do find yourself bonking, the quickest way to right yourself again is by downing a Coke or similar beverage, though this is mostly just a patch and you should ride within yourself and seek proper nutrition and recovery as soon as possible.

RIDING WITH OTHERS

Group rides are one of the more enjoyable aspects of road cycling. When all goes smoothly, riding in a pack is like being part of a flock of migrating birds. Plus, the shelter of your fellow riders means you'll be able to ride steadily at speeds you couldn't maintain on your own.

However, when familiarizing yourself with the act of road riding, you should start out either alone or with just one or two partners. This will give you ample opportunity to familiarize yourself with your bicycle as well as to assess your own physical abilities without feeling pressured to keep up with more experienced riders. Most important, riding in a group requires both skill and experience, and if you cause a crash you'll be branded with the epithet "squirrelly rider."

While your first solo rides should be enjoyable above all else, here are some skills to work on if you plan to one day introduce yourself to polite road cycling society:

• **Holding your line.** This means keeping your bike straight, which might seem obvious, but if you're a new cyclist your bike is probably weaving like a seamstress at a loom. Not only is weaving a waste of energy, but it's also liable to cause a crash in a group riding situation.

To test your line-holding skills, see if you can ride along a painted line in the road like it's a balance beam. (Only do this when it's not raining; those painted lines are slippery when wet.) You may be surprised at how difficult this is. Now, keep in mind that in a tight pack the nearest rider's wheel may be mere centimeters from yours. This is why line-holding is important: touching wheels is a sure way to crash.

Remember: Riding in a straight line is like carrying a tray full of cocktails. You want to make sure to look ahead of you, because if you focus too intently on the cocktails, they're going to spill.

Also, it's not enough to hold your line while looking forward. Remember how your bike "goes where you look"? A look to the side or over your shoulder will cause you to drift, in which case you could easily take out half the pack. So don't ride in a big group until you can turn your head and still hold your line.

• **Climbing.** While torturous, climbing can also be one of the more sublime aspects of road riding. Climbing requires rhythm and focus, and therefore leaves little room for what the Buddhists call "monkey mind," or what the rest of us call "bullshit." At its best, it is meditative and contemplative. It also builds fitness, both physical and mental.

When it comes to your climbing technique, there are no rules except this: *Do whatever you need to in order to reach the top.* Every climb is different, and every rider is different. Shift as often or as little as you like. You may want to alternate between standing and sitting in order to employ different muscle groups. You may want to stay out of the saddle and stomp your way up or you may want to sit and grind away. Slide back on the saddle for leverage or slide forward to get over the pedals. Whatever works for you.

Climbing is also another situation in which you will probably find yourself weaving or drifting if you're not careful, which is dangerous because when the pack's spread out on the big climb and everyone's got their heads down, the last thing anybody needs is you knocking them over. Be aware of your surroundings.

||||||||||||||||||||||

COPING WITH SPEED WOBBLE

Some riders are afflicted by a highly disconcerting phenomenon commonly known as "speed wobble," wherein the bicycle begins to shimmy at high speed like an aircraft breaking apart as it approaches the sound barrier. Many factors can contribute to speed wobble, such as:

• RIDER NERVOUSNESS

When you're riding a bicycle you're a vital part in a circuit consisting of the road, your bicycle, and you. The road surface sends signals through your bicycle, which in turn transmits them to your body. You then absorb those signals and return them to the bike in the form of rider input. In order for this circuit to function properly, you need to be relaxed and loose—even on searingly fast eye-watering descents. If you stiffen up, you short out the circuit and the bike can start to wobble as a result.

• RIDER POSITION

If you feel your bike start to wobble at high speed, position your pedals parallel to the road surface and close your knees together around the top tube. This can help stabilize the bike and give you better control. Also, shift more of your weight over the front wheel by moving your hands to the drops (which is where they should be anyway).

• WHEEL AND TIRE IMPERFECTIONS

Spin both wheels and look for wobbles. If your wheel is out of true, you may not notice it in most riding conditions, but it may be enough to induce speed wobble at high speeds. The same goes for your tire casing if it is bulging or otherwise inconsistent.

• BEARING PLAY

Loose headset bearings can throw your bike's handling into disarray, as can loose hub bearings, so make sure there's no excessive play anywhere on your bike.

• FRAME GEOMETRY

Sometimes speed wobble can be an accident of bike design, frame geometry, and component choice. Larger bikes, for example, tend to be more prone to it—at least anecdotally. If you suspect this to be the case, first rule out the above factors, then experiment with your bike fit. Try lowering your bars or switching to a longer stem. Wider tires and lower air pressure can also make your bike handle more confidently, as can lowering your saddle and moving it back slightly. Long and low is best when it comes to descents.

Climbing feels Sisyphean enough without drifting newbies introducing entropy into the equation.

Don't drift unpredictably, but do use the entire road (or as much of it as you can without riding into oncoming traffic), because some parts of the road are steeper than others. For example, if a turn is slightly banked, you may save a bit of energy by approaching it from the outside, which is the shallowest part of the road, and moving to the inside.

• **Descending.** What goes up must come down, and a long descent is your reward after a difficult climb. Now, you probably got pretty hot on that climb, which means you may have unzipped your jersey or removed gloves and various layers. Zip up and put everything back on again before you start descending, because you're going to get cool again in the wind and you don't want to fuss with that stuff at high speed.

Remember the braking instructions earlier. Descending in the drops will make you more aerodynamic and give you more braking power. If you can't remain in your drops, then your bars are set too low. Keep your elbows and knees tucked in for better aerodynamics. Brake *before* going into a turn. Scan the road surface for irregularities (and those damn armadillos). Keep an eye on the road shoulder—you never know when a deer will leap out of the brush or when you'll meet the rear end of a stalled automobile. Look as far down the road as possible; if you don't know what's coming up ahead, *slow down.* Look out for oncoming drivers cutting the corners, and watch the brake lights of the drivers ahead of you.

• **Sprinting.** Sooner or later you're going to want to mix it up in the town line sprint on the group ride. *Do not* attempt to sprint against another cyclist until you can sprint by yourself without deviating from your line. *Do not deviate from your line!* You must keep your front wheel planted on the road surface at all times. Sprint

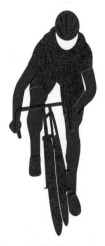

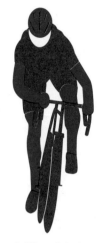

Sprinting in the drops. Sprinting on the hoods.

in the drops for maximum leverage and control. Do not sprint in the hoods, and *definitely* do not sprint with your hands on the bar tops. It's fine to rock your bike from side to side for leverage, but if you overdo it your front wheel might flop out from under you, causing you to crash. Commit to the sprint! *Do not* change your mind and stop suddenly while sprinting, or the person on your wheel will crash into you. *Do not* sprint against people who do not realize they're involved in a sprint. *Do not* sprint when you're fatigued—if you are feeling tired and sloppy, you have no business mixing it up in a sprint. Most important, if you somehow manage to win a sprint, *do not give a victory salute* unless there's an audience and it's a national championship of some kind. Otherwise you look ridiculous.

• **Riding no-handed.** There's absolutely nothing wrong with stopping to eat, checking your phone, or shedding a layer of clothing, but once you start riding in a group you're not always going to have the luxury of doing that without getting dropped, so you need to learn how to do that stuff on the bike—and without taking everybody out. Plus, sometimes it's helpful to stretch out a bit on a long ride. So get used to simple no-handed tasks like reaching into your jersey pockets, peeling a banana, and removing your gloves. These things should become second nature, and you should be able to do them while holding that all-important line.

• **Minute speed adjustments.** When riding in a group, you may need to slow down in order to avoid touching wheels with the rider ahead of you. However, if you slow down too quickly you'll take out the rider behind you. If possible, try slowing down without using the brakes. You can do this simply by sitting up and letting wind resistance do its job. If that doesn't work, feather your rear brake—a flick or two of the lever should be enough to slow you down without taking the rider behind you by surprise. If neither of these things is possible, signal and pull out of the pack. Then, blow your nose, stretch, make whatever adjustments you need to, and hop onto the rear of the pack.

• **Bunny hopping.** Swerving for road obstacles is a sure way to cause a crash, so you need to be able to hop them. No, you don't need to be able to jump over a Volkswagen, but you should be able to hop your bike over a small pothole or road seam without changing direction.

ETIQUETTE

Roadies are a fussy bunch. It's not enough just to not crash into them. They expect all kinds of other niceties from you, too. Such as:

• **Pointing out obstacles.** When riding in a group, you should always point out potholes, glass, and other hazards to the rider behind you so they're not taken by surprise. You may occasionally want to verbally warn the group of things like approaching cars. ("Car back!" "Car up!" And so forth.) However, you should do so sparingly, because there's always someone with a hair trigger who calls out every single thing they see ("Leaf up!" "Empty potato chip bag back!" And so forth), and you do not want to be that rider.

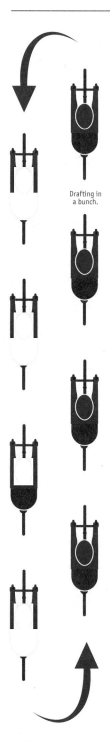

Drafting in a bunch.

• **Not being a wheelsucker.** You're just riding along and you see a Lycra-clad speck on the horizon, so to test yourself you put your head down and attempt to close the gap. Once you've succeeded, you latch on to the rider's wheel, sit up, and enjoy the ride while you catch your breath.

Do not do this.

There are few things more disconcerting or irritating than picking up a freeloader in your slipstream. The sudden materialization of another rider behind you means now you've got to worry about them not crashing into you if you need to slow down and all the rest of it—and that's if you even realize they're there in the first place, because some wheelsuckers will quietly latch on to you like pilot fish and sit there for miles before you notice them.

It's fine to use another rider as your race hare, but when you catch them either follow at a polite distance or pass them and be on your way.

• **Polite passing.** Speaking of passing, when you do so your body language is important. Passing someone closely and then looking over your shoulder at them as you sprint away says, "You want some of this?"—and in almost every case, the answer is no.

On the other hand, giving someone a wide berth as you pass and then flashing a friendly wave says, "I'm not trying to show off or engage you in competition. I'm merely acknowledging we happen to be traveling at different speeds." If real estate on the road is tight you might want to give them a polite warning as well. (A ring of the bell if you have one or else a chipper "Coming through on your left" will do nicely. Don't shout *on your left* urgently; it is rude and you will come off as a total tool.)

• **Waving.** Some cyclists feel very strongly that you should always wave to oncoming cyclists, and they consider any failure to do so tantamount to an insult.

Come on.

If you're one of these cyclists, you should temper your expectations. In fact, it is every rider's choice whether or not to wave. Waving also depends on the circumstances, so you should base your decision on the following:

—Do you feel like it?

If you're happy, wave. If you're not happy, don't wave. As long as you don't flip somebody off, you're acting within the parameters of civilized society.

—Town or country?

Are you in a busy place? Are there cyclists everywhere? If so, it's kind of silly to wave at all of them like you're running for office.

Conversely, if you're on a country lane and you encounter the first cyclist you've seen in the past hour, then a wave is probably warranted. If nothing else it's an acknowledgment that you're there for each other in an emergency—assuming it arises during the two-second window you're in close proximity to each other.

—Did they wave first?

If someone waves at you first this puts you in the uncomfortable position of having to return the wave or else come off as rude. If this bothers you but you don't want to snub them entirely, you may want to consider a waving alternative, such as a begrudging nod or a perfunctory finger lift without removing your hand from the bars.

—Is it safe?

Sometimes it's simply not practical to take your hands off the bars—like on rough terrain, for instance. Are you supposed to risk crashing and breaking your jaw for some dubious social convention? Of course not. If someone needs a wave that badly they have deeper issues and should seek professional help.

—*Other vehicles?*

Motorcyclists will occasionally wave at cyclists. It's touching when this happens, because it's an acknowledgment that we're all two-wheeled siblings, even those of us who ride farty Harley-Davidsons.

Because a wave from a motorcyclist is kind of special, you should always return it if possible. Keep in mind that motorcyclists do a funny low wave where they hold their hand downward like they're letting a puppy smell it.

It is unlikely you will encounter a motorist who waves to you out of sheer friendliness, but if you do, you are under no obligation to acknowledge the wave or return it. You owe these people nothing.

WET CONDITIONS

• Ride slower and give yourself plenty of stopping time. Not only is the road surface more slippery, but if you're using rim brakes it takes a few wheel rotations to clear the water off the rim, so you'll want to account for that.

• Lower your tire pressure a bit. This will give you better traction because more of the tire will be in contact with the road.

• Conditions are most treacherous just as a light rain starts falling on dry pavement, because it mixes with all the oil residue on the road surface and becomes extremely slippery. Take extra care.

• If it's below freezing, beware of black ice, which forms first on bridges and overpasses.

• Nearly as dangerous as black ice are metal grates, manhole covers, and painted lines, which become extremely slick in the rain.

• Rain can render your eyewear foggy and useless. A cycling cap is sometimes a better choice because the brim will protect your face and allow you to watch the road. A front fender can also help protect your face from road spray.

• If you know it's going to rain, then wear dark colors; cycling shorts become translucent when wet, and if you're wearing white, then you might as well be naked.

• Carry a PVC rain cape if it's cloudy. These fit in your jersey pocket, or even in an empty water bottle cage.

Off-Road Riding

Off-road riding (commonly referred to as "mountain biking" even though mountains are only occasionally involved) is the act of riding a bicycle on off-road trails, often in wooded areas or through parkland.

Off-road riding includes everything from riding on fire roads and singletrack to the gray area between cycling and extreme sports. If you want to put on a jersey with an energy drink logo on it and launch yourself off a ramp, then go right ahead. However, this is a book about cycling so we're going to concern ourselves more with riding and less with stunting.

When riding off-road you should first determine the ownership of the land on which you intend to ride and confirm whether or not bicycles are in fact allowed. Riding on trails that are officially closed to bicycles is called "poaching," and you should not do it. You may be the sort of rugged outlaw type who don't cotton to no signs, but there may very well be an advocacy group working hard to change the rule, and by disregarding the current rules you undermine those efforts.

The biggest challenge to road riding is drivers, whereas the biggest challenge to mountain biking is ill-behaved mountain bikers.

BE PREPARED

Once you've identified a legal trail network, you can attempt to ride on it. Make sure you take a map with you (preferably a paper one, because those don't require cell phone signals, run out of batteries, or shatter when you fall on them), and start on the trails marked beginner. Don't overestimate your abilities. Give yourself plenty of daylight in case you get lost. If possible, pick a smallish park, where if you get disoriented the worst thing that will happen is you pop out of the park and into a backyard barbecue or the parking lot of an Arby's.

It's entirely possible you might not see another cyclist during the course of your ride, and unless you're riding in Narnia there are no elves running bike shops or delis in the trunks of hollowed-out trees. Therefore, make sure you have everything you need with you: food, water, flat repair tools, and a multitool and some spare chain links. You *will* fall down at some point, so it's important to be able to make adjustments to your bike if necessary and get yourself rolling again. Hiking is pleasant, but not when you're dragging a broken bike with you.

You can't always count on getting a cell phone signal on the trail, so you can't rely exclusively on your phone like you do when it comes to every other aspect of your life. If you're riding alone, let someone know where you're going. This way, if you fall into a ravine and don't come home they'll send someone to look for you and you won't end up having to hack your own leg off with a tire lever.

SETTING UP YOUR BIKE

Prepare your bike for off-road riding. Tire pressure is perhaps the most important aspect of bike setup. If your tire pressure is too high, the tread will not conform to the trail surface and you'll experience poor traction and a bouncy ride. If your tire pressure is too low, the tire will squirm disconcertingly when you corner and possibly cause you to crash. Ignore any psi recommendations on the tire's sidewall. Instead, experiment and find the pressure that works best for you.

If your bicycle is equipped with suspension, you'll want to make sure that's adjusted properly too, because poorly adjusted or broken suspension is worse than no suspension. If the shop didn't set it up for you when you bought the bike, attempt to identify the make and model of your suspension system, consult the Internet, and follow your manufacturer's instructions. Basically, these are the two aspects you need to be most concerned about, grossly simplified:

• **Compression.** This is how squishy the suspension is. Not squishy enough and it will be too stiff over the bumps; too squishy and it will bottom out. You want to be somewhere in the middle.

• **Rebound.** After the shock compresses it returns to its normal position. If it rebounds too fast, you'll feel like you're riding a pogo stick. If it rebounds too slow, you'll feel like you're stuck in the mud. You want to be somewhere in the middle.

Don't be scared of your suspension settings. As with your tire pressure, you should experiment until you find what works best for you.

More important, don't be scared to ride a bike without suspension. You don't need it to have fun on a mountain bike, just like you don't need a home theater system to watch sitcoms on Netflix.

Suspended or not, your bike will buck around on rugged terrain, so you might also want to consider lowering your saddle slightly for better control.

BASIC SKILLS

• **Clearing obstacles.** The most fundamental mountain biking skill is riding over obstacles, something you rarely need to do when riding on pavement (save for the odd pothole or curb crossing). You need to be able to lift both your front *and* rear wheels while riding in order to clear obstacles properly. The nature of these obstacles

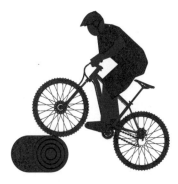 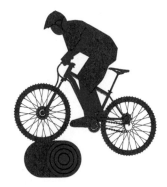

varies depending on the region, but in wooded areas the most common obstacle will be logs.

When approaching a log crossing, pop your front wheel up and place it on top of the log like you're asserting your dominance over it. Then, as your front wheel rolls over and off the log, pick up your rear wheel and hoist it over the log as well. Make sure you leave ample butt and thigh clearance for your saddle or else it might pop you in the crotch like a jackhammer as it clears the log and send you flying.

If picking up your wheels doesn't come naturally, then spend a little time practicing on a flat surface. Pretend you're surrounded by scorpions and you need to squash them one by one with your wheels. (To accelerate your learning, use real scorpions.)

You may be tempted to pick up your front wheel and then let your rear wheel simply roll over the log. This kind of lazy, sloppy riding is like dragging your heels while you walk. Plus, it can result in flat tires or crashes.

If the log is small, you may opt to simply jump over it instead. Lift the front wheel first, then follow through with the rear. This will give you more height and better control. You're a pole vaulter, not a long jumper. If you lift them both at the same time and clip the log as you sail over it you will go flying into the underbrush. Think of a horse running the steeplechase and you've got the idea.

Always know what's on the other side of the obstacle. If you

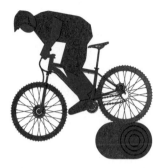
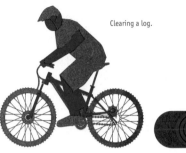

Clearing a log.

can't see what's going on, stop and check before attempting to cross. Just because some thoughtful individual built a log ramp on one side of the obstacle doesn't mean there's another one waiting for you on the other side too.

• **Climbing.** When climbing, shift your haunches over your rear wheel in order to maintain traction, and at the same time lean your shoulders forward so your front wheel stays in contact with the ground. If you're doing it right, you'll look like you're trying to scratch your ass with your rear tire and lick your front tire simultaneously.

If the climb is rocky or rooty (what mountain bike types call "technical") you'll want to get into a low gear well ahead of time so you can focus on picking your way through instead of hunting for that lower gear after it's too late. On the other hand, if the climb is relatively smooth, you may want to come into it fast and in a bigger gear so that your momentum carries you to the top.

If you lose momentum or get hung up on a steep climb you will fall over.

• **Descending.** Shift your weight back and over your rear wheel on steep descents, like you're still trying to scratch that pesky butt itch. This will keep you from going over the bars. Brake with both hands and be sure to engage your mental ABS—if your rear wheel lifts, ease up on the front brake, and if your rear wheel skids, ease up on the rear brake. Be Patrick Swayze or Demi Moore as the case may be.

• **Traversing rock gardens.** Get your elbows out, your shoulders down, and your ass back in order to keep your center of gravity low and distribute your weight as evenly as possible across the bike. Stay loose! Your bike will bounce around, but if you fight it you will lose. Keep your weight off the saddle so that the bike can move as much as it needs to, and move your own body too in order to compensate for the bike's lurching. Look for the smoothest line through and guide the bike accordingly, and together you'll find your way.

• **Negotiating ledges and drop-offs.** When riding off a ledge, get way back behind the saddle, or else when your front wheel hits you'll go right over the bars and hit the ground headfirst like a wrestler falling victim to the dreaded pile driver maneuver. If the ledge looks too high to ride off of then it is. You've got nothing to prove. If you're spooked by something just walk the bike. It beats a broken collarbone.

ETIQUETTE

• **Stay off muddy trails.** Mountain bike marketing may have given you the impression that mud is an essential component of the off-road cycling experience, and that if you don't emerge from the woods covered in filth and muck then you're not a "real" mountain biker.

This is completely untrue. Riding on wet trails causes damage to the trails in the form of ruts and erosion, so when you finish your ride covered in mud you're basically announcing that you're wildly inconsiderate and completely clueless. Basically, it's the equivalent of walking through wet cement just moments after workers have finished repaving the sidewalk, and then giving them the finger on top of it all.

The effect of rain on trails differs from region to region, season to season, and even from trail to trail. Understand the implications of heavy rainfall on your local riding spot and give trails the time they need to drain. If conditions are sloppy and you're dying to ride, stick to the road until the trails dry and firm up again.

Also, if you live someplace with a real winter, *stay off the trails in early spring*. Yes, you've been dying to ride, but the trails are at their most delicate and sensitive just after the thaw. You might as well be riding on pudding at this point.

If you're leaving an imprint of your tire tread behind you—or you're finishing the ride covered in mud—then you shouldn't be on the trails in the first place.

• **Yield when appropriate.** On the road you're "one less car," but on the trails you're an invasive species and very possibly the only machine out there. Pay attention. Don't go blasting around blind corners. People are trying to enjoy nature, and they shouldn't have to worry about getting clobbered by self-absorbed cyclists in the process. Yield to trekkers, hikers, suburban power walkers, or whichever type of human fauna is indigenous to your local trail system—and offer them a friendly greeting while you're at it.

Off-road cycling is as much about politics as anything else, because trail access for cycling is tenuous in many places. All it takes are a few noisy taxpayers to complain at the next town hall meeting for bikes to get banned forever.

If equestrians use your local trails, yield to them too, and take extra care not to scare their horses. This may seem unfair, since horses are massive snorting beasts that leave giant piles of manure all over the place, whereas bicycles are small, clean, and silent machines that are saving the world one pedal stroke at a time. However, the bond between humans and horses is something like five thousand years old, whereas bikes have only been around since the late nineteenth century, so when it comes to an entitlement face-off, the cyclist is going to lose every time.

As for your fellow cyclists, if you're heading downhill and you encounter someone heading uphill, yield to that rider. There are few things more frustrating to the off-road cyclist than *climbus interruptus*, and if you force someone off their line while they're climbing, it can be very hard for them to get going again. When passing another rider from behind, wait until the trail is wide enough, and then give the rider ahead some form of polite notice. "Mind if I slip by you on your left?" is good. "*Achtung!*" is not. Don't be a show-off, and don't be impatient. Startling a novice rider could cause them to go off the trail and crash.

- **Stay reasonably quiet.** Have some decorum. Don't whoop it up like a frat boy or sorority girl.
- **Don't ride with a sound system on your handlebars—ever.**
- **Say how many.** Whenever you encounter another trail user, regardless of their mode of transport, it's polite to let them know how many people are in your party. "It's just me," "I've got one more behind me," and so on as the case may be. This way your friend who's bringing up the rear doesn't take them by surprise. (Or they don't remain in suspense while waiting for your friend who doesn't exist.)

A WARNING ABOUT TECHNOLOGY

There is a lot of technological development in mountain biking. This is because the effects of these "advancements" are very noticeable. When a manufacturer says their new road bike wheel is more aero, you've mostly got to take their word for it. But when they introduce a new type of suspension, the effect is immediately apparent, since there's not a lot that's subjective about riding over rocks and logs—if the suspension works you'll know right away.

Unfortunately, the upshot of this constant advancement is that instead of people adapting their riding style to the terrain, riders are now adapting the terrain to themselves and their ever more technologically advanced bikes. As bikes "improve" it informs the way organizations build and maintain trails. Wheels getting big-

ALTERNATIVES TO TECHNOLOGY: RIDE SMART, NOT EXPENSIVE

• INSTEAD OF SUSPENSION, USE YOUR BODY

A little technique coupled with a high-volume tire will get you over most rough patches. Relax your arms and get out of the saddle. You may have to slow down instead of blasting your way through, but fingerpicking is more interesting than playing power chords all day.

• INSTEAD OF DROPPER POSTS, USE QUICK-RELEASE SEAT CLAMPS

The new must-have component in mountain biking is the dropper post—basically this allows you to automatically lower your saddle for the tricky spots and then raise it again on faster sections. Come on. Instead of spending over $200 on a failure-prone seat post, just install a quick-release seat clamp like they used in the old days and spend the two seconds it takes to stop and adjust your saddle—or, better yet, pick a nice halfway point for your saddle height, leave it there, and work around it. It's not that hard.

• INSTEAD OF TUBELESS TIRES, USE FINESSE

Tubeless tires allow you to run lower pressure without worrying about pinch flats, and they can also be self-sealing in the event of a puncture. At the same time, seating and sealing tubeless tires is less convenient than old-fashioned inner tubes, and while the benefits are nice, tubeless is far from a necessity if you ride with some finesse. This means paying more attention to your line and taking care to unweight when riding over obstacles—which you should be doing anyway.

• INSTEAD OF FAT BIKES, GET A LIFE

Fat bikes ostensibly allow you to ride all winter through blizzards, but there's also nothing wrong with, you know, doing something else. For every person riding a fat bike through twelve inches of snow in February there's a lonely spouse, partner, or child wondering why Mommy or Daddy (or husband or wife as the case may be) would rather be in the forest than sitting by the fire or building a snowman. Plus, snowy trails still have to be groomed for fat bikes, which means a lot of these people spend more time plowing than riding.

ger? Tires getting fatter? Suspension getting more sophisticated? Let's build bigger jumps! Let's pile the logs higher! Let's justify these upgrades!

It's the soft-tail wagging the dog. If hiking were anything like mountain biking we'd all be walking around in the woods looking like Robocop.

Moreover, the sheer pervasiveness of all this technology has given rise to the idea that it's impossible to enjoy riding off-road without a state-of-the-art mountain bike.

This is emphatically not true.

There's certainly nothing wrong with enjoying all this technology. New bike stuff is undeniably fun and exciting, and the world of off-road riding contains lots of toys to play with. At the same time, the cost of this equipment and the time and resources necessary to maintain it can be frustrating and off-putting, so it's all too easy to look at this stuff and decide it's not worth bothering with mountain biking in the first place.

Therefore, it's important to remember that you don't *need* any of this stuff. Not only is it possible to ride a simple mountain bike, but it's arguably more fulfilling. Sure, off-road cycling can be about conquering the terrain—but its essence is more about working *with* the terrain. It's perfectly fine to acknowledge that your bicycle has limits and so do you. Not every part of your bike has to be hydraulic, and not every obstacle has to be rideable the first time. Mountain bikers who start off with full-suspension bikes miss out on the fundamentals. Figuring out how to work with what you have will make you a far better rider than "upgrading" to a more "advanced" bicycle.

Lastly, whether you're riding a road bike or a mountain bike, remember: *Don't fight the bike!* This is especially important in loose terrain such as sand and gravel. Get your weight over the back wheel for traction, loosen up, and let your front wheel find its way through. If you stiffen up or fight the front wheel you're going down.

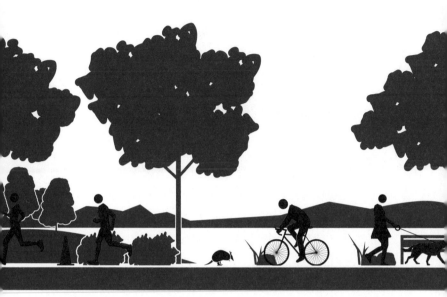

Recreational Riding on Bikeways, Greenways, and Multiuse Paths

Cycling isn't all fighting your way through city traffic, or climbing mountains in Lycra, or trundling through rock gardens on a bike with knobby tires. There's also the simple pleasure of a leisurely ride on your local car-free recreational path. However, while seemingly benign, this type of cycling can be fraught with danger—or at least considerable annoyance. Be prepared to encounter the following hazards.

RUNNERS

Cyclists and runners on multiuse trails have a lot in common: They're fitness-minded, they're looking to work out in a car-free environment, and they're partial to fanny packs.

However, cyclists and runners often come into conflict on the bike path, and indeed in the absence of their mutual enemy the car, they often turn on each other.

This is unfortunate, for we should be united in our dorky fitness goals, and the problem is often merely one of misunderstanding.

You might find runners irritating while you're cycling, but technically they're more vulnerable than you, so as the path user operating a machine, the onus is on you to anticipate their behavior and act accordingly. Therefore, you can preclude most conflicts by familiarizing yourself with the characteristics of the typical multiuse path runner:

• **Runners scare easily.** Passing a runner might seem as simple as riding past them. However, the effect of running on the human brain is profound, and it releases endorphins that cause the runner to hear the *Chariots of Fire* theme and feel like they're the only humans on Earth, no matter how crowded the path may be. Consequently, your appearance in their peripheral vision will invariably cause them to jump, possibly swerve into you, and maybe even curse you out.

To prevent this, be sure to alert runners that you're about to pass. If you have a bell, ring it. If you don't, say something like "Passing on your left." (Make sure you then actually pass on their left; you don't want to fake them out on top of everything else.) If you have a really loud hub, pedal backward so they think they're being attacked by a swarm of bees.

Unfortunately, your warning will probably be ineffective because many runners use headphones. (Presumably to drown out that cheesy *Chariots of Fire* theme.) In that case, give them plenty of room as you pass and hope for the best.

Also, remember how your bike goes where you look? The same thing happens to runners. This means that if they do turn to acknowledge your warning, they're liable to run right into you in the process. Factor this in to your passing space calculus.

• **Runners change direction suddenly.** Runners are often guided by invisible forces such as highly specific training regimens, heart rate monitors, and electronic fitness trackers. As such, it's not uncommon for a runner to simply stop running without warning

Parking the bike

When parking, don't lock your bike on top of someone else's bike, or otherwise block their access to it. Sometimes this can happen by accident—you might accidentally pass your lock through someone else's bike at a crowded rack, for example—so pay attention to what you're doing. The unwritten law (which is now official and no longer unwritten since I'm writing it in a book) is that if someone locks their bike to yours, you may extract your bike by any means necessary, including but not limited to destroying their bike.

The world does not owe you a convenient parking spot. When you ride a bike you don't have to circle the block to find parking, but the problem with this is that it's easy to become spoiled. If the bike rack is full, move on to the next one. Ultimately you may have to park your bike around the corner or—gasp!—across the street from where you're going. This is not a big deal. Don't cram your bike into a full rack where you make it difficult for everyone else to get to their bikes—or, worse, choose proximity over security, lock your bike to something flimsy, and return to find your bike gone.

due to an alert from some unseen digital apparatus, or to abruptly about-face and run in the other direction as though they just realized they forgot something important. This unpredictable behavior is a common cause of runner/cyclist collisions. So don't follow or pass them too closely, and instead treat them as you would a squirrel or rabbit—just as likely to scamper into your path as they are to halt abruptly.

• **Runners fan out.** You will often encounter groups of runners trotting three, four, and even five abreast, and the effect is a gluteal road block that can render the path totally impassible. Whatever you do, *do not attempt to breach the wall*, for the resulting confusion may cause the runners to scramble and you will go down in a maelstrom of New Balance and yoga pants. Instead, get the alpha runner's attention (there's always one; you can tell by the belt with little water bottles on it) and then verbally negotiate your way through politely yet insistently—like it's a border crossing, your passport was stolen by pickpockets, and you just wanna go home already.

DOG OWNERS

The typical suburbanite is beset by forces beyond his or her control: the overbearing boss, the rambunctious child, the incessantly running toilet in the half-bath downstairs . . . and you can add the disobedient dog to the list.

The dog owner out perambulating on the multiuse path will make a great show of their mastery over the canine as you approach. "Odin? Sit!" they boom authoritatively, indicating that you should proceed. But Odin the bichon frise has other plans, and thanks to that twenty-foot retractable leash (or complete lack of a leash) he has plenty of time to overtake you and sink his tiny little teeth into your calf before you're able to sprint away.

Unless it's a certified seeing-eye dog or a German shepherd under the command of an actual Navy SEAL, assume that every dog is liable to do whatever the hell it wants, and that its owner is mostly powerless to stop it.

OTHER CYCLISTS

While racing unwitting cyclists is inappropriate in any situation, it's especially egregious on the multiuse path, which you should consider a demilitarized zone when it comes to spirited riding. This is a place where all sorts of people come together to enjoy car-free recreation, from children to the elderly to the juggling unicyclist. Treating the recreational path as a racetrack is like graphically describing sex acts in public—bad enough anywhere, but especially so at Chuck E. Cheese's.

Nevertheless, you can be sure you'll encounter riders who think the recreational path is the testing ground for their own personal land speed record, and who weave and wheel suck their way through power walkers and children on training wheels. The most fearsome of these riders is the triathlete, readily identifiable by their aerobars and teardrop helmet. Triathletes are unpredictable bike handlers in any context (they ride more like runners than cyclists), but they're at their worst on the recreational path, where they're like a cat trying to get out of a bathtub. So avoid them whenever possible, and if one ends up on your wheel like toilet paper on your heel, just peel off and wave them through.

PEDESTRIANS

Yield to pedestrians. Yes, they will cross against the light. Yes, they will step out mid-block from between parked cars. Yes, they will walk around in a daze, as though their smartphones are emitting a tractor beam and dragging them around by the face. Still, they're the more vulnerable road user, so it's up to you to be alert. Deal with it. Consider it *noblesse oblige.*

If you're attentive and riding at a reasonable speed, you shouldn't have trouble avoiding even the most hopelessly oblivious pedestrians.

YOUR PLACE IN SOCIETY

Okay, we've arrived at Chapter 5. By now you own a bike, you ride a bike, and you're reading a book about bikes.

Guess what?

You're officially a cyclist.

You may not have an official certificate that says as much, but you probably have at least one pair of Lycra shorts and a grease stain on your pant leg—and you may even be contemplating a bicycle-themed tattoo (Don't do it!!!)—so that's pretty much the same thing.

Now that you're a cyclist, you may choose to involve yourself in matters of cycling advocacy, or you may prefer to keep to yourself. Either is fine. After all, some people are drawn to cycling for the sense of community, whereas others value the solitude and opportunities for contemplation it provides. Some even enjoy both.

Still, like it or not, as a cyclist you now occupy a certain place in society. Therefore, it's crucial to understand the implications of your newfound identity.

The mere act of pedaling a bicycle can be provocative, because it sends shock waves through certain precincts in our culture. Most important, while cycling itself is an inherently benign act, you always ride with the specter of your own mortality, for at times it can be a matter of life and death.

YOUR RIGHTS AS A CYCLIST

People like to say that cyclists have the same rights and responsibilities as drivers.

You'll hear this one a lot, and it's pretty catchy.

Unfortunately, in practice it's completely untrue.

Drivers have the benefit of a vast interstate highway system that's set aside just for them. They're also far more insulated from the consequences of their own mistakes (or those of others), both physically, by the vehicle in which they're driving, and also by administrative protections such as insurance. There is also an undeniable pro-driver bias in our society because driving is the default mode of transportation for so many people.

Cyclists, if they're lucky, sometimes get a bike lane. If a driver hits you because they drifted into the bike lane while texting, you'll find out just how much physical and administrative protection you have as a nondriver. Not enough. The driver's insurance company might help you out, but only after grilling you about whether or not you were wearing a helmet.

The Myth of Equality

It's essential to the automotive industrial complex (auto companies, insurance companies, oil companies, and the governments they lobby) to maintain the notion that bikes and cars are the same, even though they're vastly different by any metric, especially the laws of both chemistry and physics. Cars weigh thousands of pounds, reach highway speeds in seconds, and usually burn gasoline. Your bike weighs about twenty pounds, tops out at about twenty-five miles per hour unless you're heading downhill, and its most noxious emission is its rider's farts.

The reason that municipalities promulgate this myth is that when cars and bikes are deemed ostensibly "equal," it's far easier to deny cyclists special consideration. "Hey, you've got the same rights and responsibilities as drivers," the argument goes. "What more do you want? Bike lanes?!?" Now get out there and "share the road" with vehicles that weigh one hundred times more than yours!

Theft of the Roads

It's also crucial to remember that, about one hundred years ago, the auto industry stole the public roadways from us. In the early days of the automobile, the streets still belonged to everybody, and the assumption was that the user operating the largest, most powerful machine should yield to more vulnerable road users, which is to say everybody else. In 1908 the Model T hit the roads, and by the end of the 1920s drivers of the Tin Lizzy had killed more than two hundred thousand people. Cities moved to regulate automobiles, and the auto industry countered with lobbying and public relation campaigns, which included the notion of the "jaywalker," which was created from whole cloth. This invention was quite a coup to the auto industry, for it cemented this new concept of the victim as a bumbling idiot.

Within a generation, the roads went from being for everybody to being for cars only. Even though our roadways are still ostensibly public, you only really have full use of them if you're willing or able to buy or lease a car. As for walking on them, you really only get to do that during those precious few moments when you have the "walk" signal. Most chillingly, the appropriation of the roads comes at an enormous cost in human lives. In the United States more than thirty thousand people are killed in motor vehicle crashes every year.

If plane crashes killed anywhere near that many people, airplanes would be grounded.

Clawing Back Your Little Sliver of Tarmac Out from Under the Four Wheels of Tyranny

In recent years people have begun to realize that there's just not enough room for all these cars anymore, especially in cities, so lately we've been seeing a "return to the bike."

Unfortunately, the last three-quarters of a century of car dependency have made a real mess of things from a human perspective, so the reintegration of space for both cyclists and pedestrians does not always go smoothly. To address this, most forward-thinking cities have been making a genuine attempt to install some sort of bike and pedestrian infrastructure, which makes the streets demonstrably safer for all users. On top of this, there have been attempts in some places to wrest back some of the legal rights we've forfeited to motorists, who are often virtually immune from prosecution. For example, in New York City there's something known as the "Right of Way Law," which makes it a misdemeanor for a motorist to hit a pedestrian or cyclist who has the right of way.

(You'd think it would *always* have been a crime to hit somebody with the right of way, but you'd be wrong, which underscores just how successful the automotive industrial complex's appropriation of the roads has been. Essentially, they've succeeded in creating an environment in which drivers have almost no accountability, and where all the responsibility—and guilt—has been shifted on to the more vulnerable road users.)

In order to maintain their control of the roads, the automotive industrial complex must do all it can to make sure drivers are absolved of responsibility. This is why they love to tell cyclists to wear helmets. It's the easiest way of making safety entirely *your responsibility*, and campaigns telling you to wear one have the dual benefit of making it look like the complex cares about you. After all, telling you to wear a plastic hat of dubious effectiveness is a lot easier than modernizing infrastructure for everyone's protection or returning to the notion of motorist accountability.

Your helmet Miranda rights

1. You have the right to wear a helmet, until such time as we pass a law forcing you to wear a helmet.

2. Failure to wear a helmet will be used against you in a newspaper article, regardless of its relevance. ("The cyclist's leg was severed by the drunk driver. She was not wearing a helmet.")

3. You have a right to wear a helmet while being questioned after a collision, if only to stop people from asking, "So, were you wearing a helmet?"

4. If you cannot afford a helmet, a big bulky one-size-fits-all one will be provided to you during a Free Helmet Day! sponsored by your local department of transportation or bike advocacy group. You will never wear it because it fits awkwardly and looks like a giant marshmallow.

5. You can decide not to wear a helmet, but if you do, then everything is automatically your fault.

THE RIGHTS YOU ACTUALLY HAVE

The automotive industrial complex conspiracies aside, unless you're reading this in someplace like North Korea, you've still got your basic human rights, even when you're riding a bicycle.

But let's take a look at the unwritten rights you have as a cyclist, whether anyone else likes them or not.

Entitlement

People like to say cyclists have a keen sense of entitlement. Damn right we do! Our bikes cause negligible wear and tear on the infrastructure, they take up little room when parked, they're rarely fatal to pedestrians, and they don't need a complex fueling network—unless you count Chipotle, since we do need to eat.

You can't say that about your Hyundai.

In exchange for treading lightly on the Earth, all we ask is that drivers take a little care not to run us over, and we feel perfectly comfortable with this level of entitlement. Unfortunately, not everybody agrees. Not only are many drivers unwilling to pay attention, but they've also totally remade the streets in their image, so what is a cyclist supposed to make of a typical intersection?

Sure, you've got "all the same rights and responsibilities of a driver," but queuing up in a turning bay on a busy suburban avenue while riding a bike runs counter to pretty much every survival instinct you have.

Cyclists' Bill of Rights

1. YOU HAVE THE RIGHT TO STAY ALIVE

This is the big one. Staying alive in an indifferent or outright hostile environment overrides car-centric laws and infrastructure. Breaking laws for thrills is stupid; bending laws for survival is occasionally necessary and sometimes even unavoidable.

2. YOU HAVE THE RIGHT TO THE ROADS

Drivers think they own the roads because they "pay for them." This is a myth. We all pay for them. In fact, cyclists arguably pay more than drivers since we all pay taxes yet bikes are so much kinder on the infrastructure. You know when you go out to dinner with a bunch of people and you all split the bill? Drivers are the ones who order wine, cocktails, and the big entree; you're the one who had the hummus appetizer and some ice water. Furthermore, the bike boom predates the proliferation of the automobile, and many roads were first paved with cyclists in mind. They're your roads too (and they were your roads first), and don't let anybody forget it.

3. YOU HAVE A RIGHT TO DRIVE TOO IF YOU WANT

Just because you're a cyclist doesn't mean you have to swear off driving. Indeed, depending on where you live, going car free can be a difficult or nearly impossible proposition. Practicality trumps politics and you've got to get around. Plus, let's not forget that cars are, when used responsibly, pretty damn amazing. If you need to drive, so be it.

However, be advised that if you do own or lease a car, you do forfeit all rights to display that "One Less Car" sticker.

4. YOU HAVE THE RIGHT TO A SMUG SENSE OF SUPERIORITY

It's an unavoidable by-product of riding. Enjoy it. Just keep it to yourself.

The fact is that sometimes the safest way through the intersection isn't necessarily the legal way. For example, there are circumstances in which getting a jump on the green light can give you a crucial head start against the rabid motor vehicle pack behind you. The trick is you've got to know when law bending is safe and appropriate and when it's not, and this only comes with experience. Nevertheless, in cycling, the letter of the law might as well be written in a different alphabet.

YOUR RESPONSIBILITIES AS A CYCLIST

1. Be considerate to pedestrians. Remember how the auto industry stole the streets from us? Well, before automobiles took over, we were the biggest menace on the road, terrorizing horses and innocent hoop-rolling children with our gigantic penny farthings.

When you factor drivers out of the equation, this is still the case, and your swiftness and stealth mean you're liable to torpedo a pedestrian if you're not mindful of them at all times. Momentum is addictive on a bicycle, so stopping can seem almost counterintuitive, but that doesn't excuse you from yielding.

It won't kill you to put a foot down now and again, but if you're unwilling to do so, you might really hurt someone else.

When a pedestrian has the right of way (which is most of the time), you give it to them. When they're in the crosswalk, they go first, not you. Don't sneak up on them—ride with traffic, not against it. Accept that pedestrians will jaywalk and ride accordingly. Get off the sidewalk. When riding in crowded public spaces, such as parks, ride slowly and considerately and pick your way through like the interloper you are.

Be considerate. Don't push your way through crowds. One of the great things about bikes is you can hop off and go into "pedestrian mode" whenever you need to. Don't beat them, join them.

2. Be considerate to drivers. Sometimes you're wrong and the driver is not. Ride predictably, signal your intentions on busy streets, and don't force law-abiding drivers (yes, they're out there) to stop short or otherwise put them into a position where they have to avoid killing or maiming you. It makes them angry, and if there's one thing drivers resent, it's having to pay attention.

New cyclists can be anxious and see danger where it doesn't exist, so don't be the petulant rider who flies into a rage at every perceived slight. Let drivers pass you when it's safe and convenient for you to do so. Yes, in many places you are entitled to the entire lane, which you should use when you need it, but don't obstruct a driver's path just because.

3. Strive for self-sufficiency. Understand the basics of your bicycle and of cycling. Maintain your bike. Lock your bike. Be prepared. Stay informed. Keep up on the local cycling news. Uphold the spirit of collective independence that makes cycling great.

This doesn't mean you shouldn't pay someone to repair your bike if you need to, and it doesn't make you an outlaw, but it does

The politics of helping

You must offer to help a fellow cyclist when it is reasonable to do so. When is it unreasonable? This is highly subjective, but you are probably within your rights to deny assistance under any one of the following circumstances:

• Taking the time to help will result in serious consequences for you (e.g., getting fired, getting in trouble with domestic partner, missing the birth of a firstborn child, etc.)

• The cyclist is rude or overly demanding

• The cyclist is in need of a tool or a pump they neglected to carry and they expect you to perform the labor for them while they lounge on the curb live-tweeting the whole thing

• The cyclist's equipment is so insanely expensive that they can clearly afford to be picked up in a helicopter

mean that as a marginalized road user, you need to adopt a survivalist mind-set.

4. Offer help to fellow cyclists in need. You're not obligated to wave to your fellow cyclists, but you are beholden to them when it comes to roadside assistance. If you come across a stranded cyclist, you must stop and offer whatever help you reasonably can.

5. Don't mess it up for everyone else. Don't poach the trails. Don't annoy pedestrians. Don't do all the stuff stupid anticycling newspaper columnists love to say cyclists do, like riding on sidewalks and harassing children and the elderly while foaming at the mouth.

6. Be modest. Riding a bicycle is a sublime pursuit and as close as you can get without leaving the ground to the sensation of flying. However, it's important not to lose sight of two things: (1) Riding a bike is so simple that even a three-year-old can do it, so get over yourself already; (2) there are people who have been doing it way, way longer than you, so don't think you know everything. Be content to be just another person on a bike.

GETTING HASSLED BY THE MAN, AND WHAT TO DO ABOUT IT

Sooner or later it's going to happen: You're going to get a ticket.

You may deserve this ticket. For example, perhaps you ran a red light at a busy intersection at full speed and caused a five-car pileup.

You also may not deserve this ticket. For example, a whiny resident may be complaining to the local precinct about "those crazy bikers," and so now you're getting a ticket for not wearing a helmet and for not riding in the bike lane, neither of which are illegal. (Well, in New York City they're not.)

Either way, you want to get through the encounter as smoothly as possible. Riding away with a ticket is better than taking a ride in a police car. Make sure you carry ID with you at all times while riding. Be polite, even if you're angry. Find out what you did wrong. If the officer's wrong, go ahead and point it out (politely), but it's probably not going to make a difference.

If it's a BS ticket, you're just going to have to fight it later.

Of course, it's always better not to get stopped at all. Ride smart. Pay attention. Follow the local bike media so you know when the crackdowns are in effect.

Chapter 6

CYCLING SUBCULTURES

I t's a fundamental truth that the more objectively silly a group of people is, the more seriously they take themselves. Consider, for example, the guards in front of Buckingham Palace, stoic and unflappable despite their adorably fuzzy Chewbacca hats.

This paradox also applies to cyclists. They, too, wear funny clothes and follow arcane rules that have little relevance in the context of the outside world. There also seems to be a direct relationship between the amount of expensive specialized equipment a cyclist owns and how humorless she is. The dude in jeans puttering around town on an old beach cruiser projects an aura of relaxed good cheer, whereas the roadie rocketing by on a $10,000 plastic race bike while wearing an adult Lycra onesie radiates disdain and scowls like Mussolini.

You may find this intimidating. Don't. Yes, some cyclists can be judgmental, but this is usually because they're in that awkward phase between "newbie" and "enlightened." When it comes to adhering to the dogma of cycling, newbies don't know any better and enlightened cyclists don't care; it's the overzealous fundamentalists who take it all too seriously.

TYPES OF CYCLISTS

Cycling is essentially a collection of subcultures and/or marketing niches that are constantly breaking apart and reforming again as bikes and riding styles come in and out of fashion, and riders switch identities and allegiances to keep up with the trends.

Subcultures you're liable to come across include but are by no means limited to:

- Road riding and racing
- Gravel grinding
- Randonneuring
- Cycle touring
- Cyclocross
- BMX
- Triathlon*
- Recumbent riding
- Urban cycling
- Alley cat racing
- Fixed-gear criterium racing
- Mountain biking
- Freeriding
- Downhilling
- Enduro
- Singlespeeding
- Bikepacking
- Commuting
- Advocacy
- Messengering, food delivery, and other forms of work cycling
- Tall bikers, outlaw bike clubs, etc.

Pigeonholing people is fun, but for scientific purposes it's largely useless to categorize cyclists according to their subculture, because the boundaries between them are both ever-shifting and highly porous. For example, a mature rider might begin the season as a roadie and end it as a cyclocross racer, with periods of commuting, mountain biking, and advocacy in between.

---

*Only qualifies as cycling one-third of the time, and even then just barely.

Feel free to take part in as many or as few cycling subcultures as you choose. Think of them as classes at the University of Cycling—you should add and drop them as often as you like, and the size of your course load is entirely at your discretion.

As for identifying other riders, instead of doing so by subculture, it's far more useful to do so based on where they are on the road to Cycling Enlightenment.

THE ROAD TO ENLIGHTENMENT

• **Beginner or "newbie."** The rider has recently obtained a bicycle. He or she may display certain distinguishing marks indicating that they have little idea what they're doing, including chainring tattoos or helmet hair. With every pedal stroke, the beginner is unwittingly committing sins that make more experienced riders cringe. Some of these sins are dangerous (weaving in a pace line or slamming on their brakes), whereas others are completely benign (wearing a "World Champion" jersey).

• **Froglet.** The rider is just beginning to find his or her legs, while developing strength and stamina. While he or she may be experimenting with clipless pedals, the Froglet is also becoming self-aware and may begin to manifest behavior that indicates curiosity of the greater cycling ecosystem, such as ordering a pair of socks or a water bottle sporting the logo of a popular bike blog.

• **Adolescent.** The rider now identifies fully as a cyclist. He or she may also identify strongly with a particular subculture, to the point of questioning the legitimacy of other subcultures or rejecting them outright. Brand names and equipment are important signifiers during this stage. The cyclist is insufferable and irritating, and inexplicably proud of physical cosmetic defects such as road rash and tan lines.

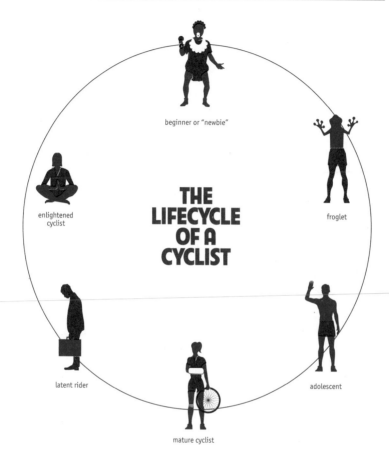

THE LIFECYCLE OF A CYCLIST

beginner or "newbie"

froglet

enlightened cyclist

adolescent

latent rider

mature cyclist

• **Mature cyclist.** During adolescence, riders face various monomythic challenges: crashes, stolen bicycles, getting dropped from the peloton in races, getting lost, and bonking in the middle of nowhere. They also face temptation in the form of other lifestyle choices, such as motorcycling, oenophilia, and golf. Riders who survive adolescence without defecting to other lifestyles become mature cyclists who are resolute in their identity yet more accepting of other cyclists.

• **Latent rider.** External demands such as family and career can result in a latency period during which the cyclist's desire or ability to ride goes dormant. This may be accompanied by weight gain and mild depression. Bike commuting and errand running are increasingly recognized by this rider as important tools for mitigating or counteracting the withdrawal symptoms that characterize the latency period.

• **Enlightened cyclist.** The enlightened cyclist is able to derive joy and fulfillment from any type of cycling, and is largely free from worldly concerns such as aesthetics, mileage, fitness metrics, riding style, or equipment choice. Enlightened cyclists can ride intensely, yet they undergo prolonged periods of not riding with little or no withdrawal symptoms, and they can be seen smiling while riding even the most unwieldy and cumbersome bicycles, such as bike-share bikes.

WHO'S LAUGHING AT YOU, WHY THEY'RE LAUGHING, AND WHY YOU SHOULD BE LAUGHING AT THEM INSTEAD

Riders who are outwardly judgmental of other cyclists are generally stuck in the middle phases of the Lifecycle of the Cyclist. Of these cyclists, some are worse than others. Here are some of the most egregious offenders.

WHO'S LAUGHING AT YOU

Roadies

WHY THEY'RE LAUGHING

Oh, please, take your pick:
- Your jersey's too big.
- Your shorts are too small.
- Your socks are too short.
- Your legs are too hairy.
- Your saddlebag is too voluminous.
- Your smile is too broad.

WHY YOU SHOULD BE LAUGHING AT THEM INSTEAD

While roadies are ostensibly laughing at your alleged sartorial errors, it's only because they're profoundly uptight, and what they're really laughing at is the fact that you're enjoying yourself, which is sad. This is because roadies don't ride; they "train." To that end, they hire coaches who tell them what to do, and if they work really hard, they get to join amateur racing teams sponsored by local dental practices. (Though they still have to pay for the uniforms, race entry fees, traveling expenses, and tooth cleanings.) Also, roadies don't have friends; they have "training partners," because they're not allowed to ride with people who are on different training programs—and even if they were, nobody would want to ride with them anyway.

So who's laughing now?

WHO'S LAUGHING AT YOU

Mountain bikers

WHY THEY'RE LAUGHING

Your bike doesn't have enough bouncy stuff on it, and you just fell down.

WHY YOU SHOULD BE LAUGHING AT THEM INSTEAD

For all their "gnar" this and "shred" that, mountain bikers are highly pampered. In fact, with the possible exception of recumbent riders, who are literally reclining while riding, no cyclists coddle themselves with their equipment more than mountain bikers do. That's why they're always bragging about how "plush" their bikes are.

Another fun fact about mountain bikers: A lot of them ride chairlifts to the top of mountains instead of riding their bikes to the top. It's true! In fact, between driving to the park and riding the lift to the top of the hill, there's not a lot of difference between mountain biking and a visit to Six Flags. These are usually the types who are laughing at you.

Mountain bikers who actually pedal their bikes on the trails generally don't laugh at other mountain bikers, because they understand riding off-road is challenging, and they know that if you're doing it right, you're bound to fall at least once.

WHO'S LAUGHING AT YOU
Recumbent riders

WHY THEY'RE LAUGHING
They're laid back and comfortable; whereas you're cutting off blood flow to your genitals as you impale your crotch on your "wedgie." (They actually call upright bicycles wedgies.)

WHY YOU SHOULD BE LAUGHING AT THEM INSTEAD
Come on, just look at them!*

WHO'S LAUGHING AT YOU
People on Dutch bikes

WHY THEY'RE LAUGHING
Like the recumbent rider, they too think that you're needlessly punishing yourself on your sporting bicycle—except instead of lying on a rolling daybed, they're sitting upright in an easy chair. They also refuse to acknowledge any bicycle that cannot be propped up on a centerstand, or that weighs less than fifty pounds.

WHY YOU SHOULD BE LAUGHING AT THEM INSTEAD
Dutch bike riders are dashing and lovely, but for all their billowy skirts, flowing scarves, and tweedy sport jackets with padded elbows, they really aren't that different from roadies in that they derive much of their self-satisfaction from their appearance and

---

* If you really are losing blood flow to your genitals, then their laughter may be justified and you should probably address that before attempting to turn the tables on them.

wardrobe. The only real difference is that the roadie is laughing at you because you're a schlub, whereas the Dutch bike rider is laughing at you because your appearance smacks of physical effort, which is antithetical to the Dutch bike ethos.

Of course, actual Dutch people who ride bikes in the Netherlands don't give any of this stuff a second thought, which is precisely what makes the non-Dutch Dutch bike rider's self-satisfaction so delightfully absurd, and why you should feel free to laugh at their pomposity and pretention.

TAKE YOUR PULLS

As you make your way through the cyclist's lifecycle, it is important to encourage those who are coming up behind you. Lend these adorable li'l wheelsuckers a metaphorical wheel for a while and help bring them up to the front of the pack. Tousle their already tousled helmet hair. Remember, you were once a complete dork too.

(In fact, you're almost certainly *still* a complete dork. We all are.)

The more smoothly we work together, the more efficient we become.

Chapter 7

COEXISTING WITH DRIVERS

Successfully navigating roadways dominated by cars is the greatest challenge you face as a cyclist, potentially surpassed only by having to endure conversations with your coworker who does triathlons. It is, however, without question, the greatest threat to your physical well-being.

It's alarming to realize that while drivers hold your life in their hands, they also hold in their hands smartphones, e-cigarettes, and pumpkin spice lattes. If this sounds scary, it's only because it is.

However, it's important to remember that drivers are not your enemy; they're simply people just like you—which is to say they're preoccupied, late, and behave incredibly selfishly at times. Yes, we're *all* selfish, and drivers are not inherently worse in this arena than cyclists. The delta is when you put us in four-thousand-pound soundproof boxes with an engine that can accelerate from zero to sixty in under ten seconds.

Cars don't change our behaviors so much as they amplify their effects. As a cyclist, you quickly come to understand this and hopefully learn to anticipate and avoid these effects when riding.

THE MOST DANGEROUS DRIVER BEHAVIORS

• **Looking right through you.** Don't rely on eye contact. Making what you think is "eye contact" with a driver doesn't mean they actually see you. Sometimes they're looking past you. Or sometimes they do see you, but they simply figure, "What the hell. I'm going to go anyway." Drivers are often confident that you will stop for them or take evasive action, even if you have the right of way.

• **Waving you through.** Occasionally a driver will stop and wave you through as a courtesy, even though they technically have the right of way themselves. They'll also act like they're doing you the biggest favor in the world, giving you a magnanimous wave like they're blessing you from the Popemobile.

They may mean well, but waving you through is dangerous, and it's important you realize this. One of the many risks is that there is another driver coming in the other direction who has no idea that you've been waved through. Unless you're absolutely sure there's nobody else coming, the best response is often, "No, *you* go. I insist."

• **Flinging the door open.** Legally speaking, in most places, if a driver opens her car door into you it's her fault—but good luck finding a driver or a police officer who will acknowledge that this is the case.

Happily cycling.

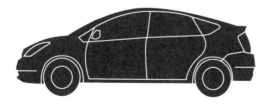
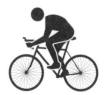

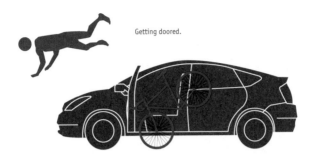

Getting doored.

You have to assume that every parked or idling car is a spring-loaded trap, and that every door you pass is liable to fly open at any moment. Also, on one-way streets, stick to the passenger-door side of the road if possible. All cars have drivers (at least for now), but not all cars have passengers, so your odds of getting doored on the passenger side of the roadway are generally slightly less.

• **Opening the door slowly, closing it, and then flinging it open again.** Once in a while you'll see a car door open slightly and then close again. You might think that the driver opened the door, checked over their shoulder, saw you coming, and closed the door again so that you could safely pass.

You would be wrong.

In fact, usually this is just a failed attempt to open the door. Don't worry, they'll do their best to get you on the second try.

• **Driving while distracted.** As a cyclist your vantage point affords you the opportunity to look into people's cars, and when you do you'll notice that many drivers are engrossed in their smartphones. Beware of these distracted drivers. If you can't actually see inside the car due to sun glare or tinted windows, you can usually identify a smartphone-addled driver by their "drift and correct, drift and correct" pattern of driving.

Another giveaway is their failure to resume driving when the light turns green, at which point everybody honks at them and then they step on the gas and fly into the intersection without looking—which is why you should *never* position yourself in front of a driver who's standing still at a green light, or run a red light because the distracted driver hasn't started driving yet.

Occasionally there are also auditory warnings. For example, thanks to hands-free systems, you may now be able to hear a driver's phone conversation from half a block away. This happens because the driver was rocking out to "Don't Stop Believin'" by Journey and then took a phone call, at which point they were already acclimatized to the high volume.

• **The pass-and-turn.** Drivers will often pass you and then, after overtaking you, turn right into your path, invariably without signaling. Unfortunately, many drivers believe they should never ever have to wait for a cyclist for any length of time or for any reason. (They expect *you* to stop for *them*, remember?) The best case is that they merely cut you off and annoy you. The worst case is what's known as a "right hook" (or left hook if the street is configured that way) and it can be deadly.

For this reason, always be aware of who's in front of you *and* who's behind you as you approach an intersection, and be ready to swerve or stop in the event a driver pounces from behind.

Most important, never overtake a driver on the inside at an intersection.

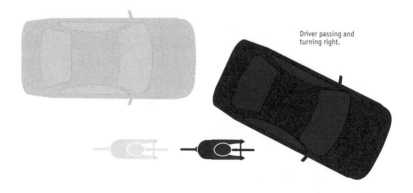

Driver passing and turning right.

• **Trawling for parking.** When looking for street parking, drivers exhibit behavior similar to that of their smartphone-addled counterparts—except instead of "drift and correct" it's "accelerate and creep, accelerate and creep."

What's especially tricky about this behavior is that both the "accelerate" and "creep" phases are arrhythmic. Therefore, you cannot predict how long a driver will creep along before suddenly rocketing down the block because they see another driver approaching a car with a set of keys in their hand and they want to get a jump on the spot.

Be extremely cautious when passing a parking trawler in the "creep phase," because they're paying attention only to the curbside, and they may decide to accelerate just as you overtake them.

• **Road rage.** You never know when a driver is going to become completely unhinged. It could be because you yelled at them for cutting you off in a classic "right hook" maneuver, or it could be because they don't like the color of your shirt.

It doesn't matter.

Typical road rage symptoms include engine revving, ranting about how you belong on the sidewalk, and threatening to get out of the car and do things to your bike and your body. *Do not engage a road rager.* Forget pride—people are freaking crazy, and too many of them have guns. Life is short enough already without some maniac shooting you. If possible, take their license plate information so that the police can fail to follow up, and then hide in the nearest Dumpster until it all blows over.

THE MOST DANGEROUS CYCLIST BEHAVIORS

Driver evasion is a vital survival skill, but don't hide behind a persecution complex and avoid responsibility for your own actions. Drivers don't have a monopoly on dangerous behavior, and there's plenty of dumb stuff you can do on a bike that can get you hurt or worse. Here are the most egregious cyclist behaviors.

• **Riding the wrong way ("salmoning").** If people are looking one way, why confound them by coming from the other direction? As a cyclist, your greatest allies are:
  1. Visibility
  2. Predictability
Salmoning confuses everybody: drivers, pedestrians, and other cyclists.

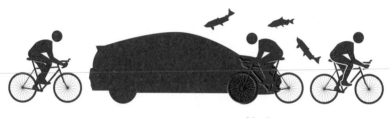

Salmoning.

• **Riding drunk.** Your bicycle is equipped with a built-in sobriety tester: If you're too drunk to ride, it falls over.

Cycling is a great alternative to driving if you want to enjoy a few adult beverages—responsibly, that is, like they tell you to do

Signs you are too drunk to ride
• You keep dropping your bike lock key.
• You're doing okay with the key but you're trying to open someone else's lock.
• You're attempting to carry a passenger whose name you don't know.
• You're attempting to carry more than one passenger, regardless of your level of familiarity.
• You have, at any point in the evening, consumed a questionable burrito or pizza slice of dubious provenance under the rationale that it will "absorb the alcohol," or you are en route to such an establishment.

in the commercials. However, just because you're a lot less likely to get pulled over and breathalyzed doesn't mean the bike is your ticket to a night of consequence-free binge drinking. Taking the bike instead of the car is smart if you want to have a couple drinks, but riding drunk is a great way to crash hard, so know your limits, and don't wait for that sobriety tester to kick in before you skip the bike and call a cab.

• **Riding while distracted.** As you get more comfortable on the bike, you may be tempted to glance at your phone while you're riding, and it's only a matter of time before you find yourself riding no-handed while texting, which is a fantastic way to hit a pothole and break your collarbone.

As far as enjoying music and other forms of auditory entertainment, laws concerning headphone use while riding vary depending on the municipality. For example, in New York City you're only allowed to ride with one headphone in, so it's a good thing the artisanal set enjoys monaural recordings along with their reclaimed wood and Edison bulbs.

Laws aside, riding while listening to music or podcasts is generally fine from a safety perspective as long as you're doing so at a sensible volume. "Sensible" means that if someone were to speak to you in a normal tone of voice you'd be able to hear them over the music. Once the volume reaches the point that you can no longer hear your environment, then it starts to become dangerous.

Many people think listening to headphones while riding is dangerous regardless of the volume, yet all cars come with very loud stereos, so go figure.

The above notwithstanding, as a cyclist you're interacting with your surroundings on a more intimate level, so keeping your ears unplugged is always the safest option.

• **Running red lights.** Speaking objectively, you should stop for all red lights, if for no other reason than it's the law.

Speaking pragmatically, running red lights while cycling is like drinking and cycling—in moderation it's not too big a deal, but if you do it egregiously it can easily kill you.

"Moderation" means stopping at the red, making absolutely sure nobody's coming, and going through—essentially treating it as a stop sign. "Egregiously" means riding straight into a busy intersection like an idiot.

• **Running stop signs.** Speaking objectively, you should come to a complete stop and put your foot down at all stop signs, if for no other reason than it's the law.

Speaking pragmatically, from a safety perspective, rolling through the stop sign is generally fine—just as long as you're going slowly enough that you can easily come to a complete stop within a foot or two, and there are no pedestrians waiting to cross.

At a four-way stop, wait your turn, just like you would in a car.

DIFFERENT TYPES OF MOTOR VEHICLES AND WHAT TO EXPECT FROM EACH
Private Vehicles

Drivers of all ages and from all walks of life who are in a really big hurry and haven't passed a road test since they were teenagers (assuming they're even licensed at all)? What could go wrong?

Potentially everything.

When interacting with motorists, prepare for the worst. Don't assume they see you or that they're going to stop for that stop sign. Don't think the bike rack or the "Keep Portland Weird" bumper sticker means they're looking out for you. Take extra care anywhere private vehicles congregate, such as shopping centers and schools. Also keep in mind that many drivers of private vehicles are cranky if not downright furious, so treat them like rabid raccoons and avoid altercations if possible.

FedEx, UPS, and Other Delivery Trucks

Take extra care when passing stopped or idling delivery trucks. First, these vehicles create blind spots for cyclists, particularly when they are parked near intersections. Second, you never know when the driver is going to appear with a hand truck, and you don't want to wind up facedown in a pile of Amazon packages. Most important, whether the truck is moving or parked, never pass it on the inside where you're trapped between the truck and the curb if you encounter an obstacle.

Taxis

Big-city taxi drivers have a bad reputation that is neither entirely deserved nor completely unwarranted. (Try driving for twelve hours at a time and see how frayed your nerves are.) When interacting with taxi drivers, the most important thing to keep in mind is that they're liable to pull over to pick up or drop off a fare at any time, so try not to find yourself between a taxi and the curb.

Far more dangerous than taxi drivers are taxi passengers, who are among the worst offenders when it comes to flinging doors open heedlessly. Weekday passengers are of the "businessperson preoccupied with the phone" variety, whereas weekend night passengers are simply drunk. Either way, they'll do their very best to "door" you into oblivion.

Pickup Trucks

Generally your biggest concern while cycling is coming into physical contact with the vehicle itself, but in the case of pickup trucks, there's also the risk of flying projectiles. Not to stereotype, but it's a rare cyclist who hasn't had something hurled at them from inside a pickup truck. Increasingly, there are also tales of pickup truck drivers who modify their exhaust systems so they can envelop cyclists and hybrid car drivers in a cloud of black smog for sport. Apparently this is called "rolling coal." Sadly, until someone develops a similar technology for bicycles—perhaps some sort of flatulence cannon—there is no way to retaliate.

Flatbed Trucks

Do not ever try to pass a flatbed truck when you are approaching an intersection. These vehicles might as well be purpose built for right-hooking you. Just because you don't see a turn signal doesn't mean the driver's not going to turn anyway.

Garbage Trucks

The municipal garbage trucks aren't so bad. Your biggest concern is slipping in garbage water. It's the private haulers you've got to watch out for—especially if you ride late at night, when they tear through the city on their rounds, running red lights in the process. Steer clear, because you don't want a visit from the boys at Barone Sanitation.

WHAT TO DO IN THE EVENT OF A COLLISION

Cycling isn't particularly dangerous. Even in North America, where motorists dominate the road, cycling is, proportionately speaking, comparable in safety to driving and walking. Odds are, if you're paying attention, you're going to be fine.

Nevertheless, there is always the possibility you might be involved in a crash with a motor vehicle—and as a cyclist in a system that favors drivers, you need to be extra vigilant in the crucial moments after the crash takes place.

Unfortunately, this is precisely when it's most difficult to be vigilant, because even if you're fortunate enough to be conscious, you've just undergone a traumatic experience and you're riddled with adrenaline.

Laws, insurance regulations, and so forth vary from place to place, but no matter where you are, it's essential to remember the following:

1. You're not fine. In the wake of that adrenaline rush, you will be awash in a profound sense of relief that you're conscious and ambulatory, coupled with a sense of embarrassment that you just fell off your bike in public. In fact, you may find yourself so elated to be alive that you brush off offers of assistance, insist you're okay, and tell the motorists to be on their way.

This is a huge mistake. You are in no state to assess your physical condition, and injuries often take some time to manifest themselves. What's more, if you let the motorist go, you could very easily find yourself with little or no recourse down the line.

2. Call 911. You'll need the police to come and take a report. Don't leave until the police have taken everybody's information, they've finished the process, and you have all the information you need to get that report at the precinct later on.

3. Find witnesses! This is huge. If anybody saw what happened, make sure you get their contact information immediately. Motorists can and will lie when making a report, and if they do, it's simply your word against theirs. If, however, you have witnesses (or video footage if you ride with a video camera on your bike), your case is that much stronger.

4. Seek medical attention. Don't be afraid of the bills. Nothing is more important than your health. Also, your hospital or doctor visit may very well be covered. For example, New York State has "no fault" laws, which means that insurance companies must pay for crash-related medical attention regardless of who was at fault.

5. Get the police report. Pick it up as soon as it's ready, but don't be surprised to find the motorist claimed you "came out of nowhere" or ran a light that you didn't. (Here's where witnesses come in handy.)

Once you've done all this, you've got a solid foundation for getting compensation for your damaged bicycle or damaged body, and you can begin the tedious process of dealing with insurance companies, lawyers, and so forth.

Chapter 8

COMPETING ON YOUR BIKE

I f you find yourself surreptitiously pacing yourself against other cyclists on your commute, picking off people one by one on charity rides, or simply obsessed with the pursuit of speed, you may be Bike Racer Positive (BR+).

Bike racing is congenital. You may discover you are BR+ at an early age, or the symptoms may lie dormant until adulthood. Either way, bike racing can be debilitating, but if you learn to channel your impulses in a positive manner, you may be able to live something resembling a normal life.

To this end, it is essential that you self-quarantine by surrounding yourself with other BR+ cyclists as much as possible. Find your local group ride. Learn how to ride in a pack. Understand what it means to trade pulls, attack, counterattack, and recover.

It's also vital that you learn to control your bike racing behavior, and that you don't foist it upon the general cycling population by wheelsucking strangers and time-trialing on the bike path while yelling, "On your left!" at toddlers on tricycles.

Fortunately for you, bike racing is a very popular sport from a participatory standpoint, and there are abundant opportunities for you to indulge your BR+ desires—though keep in mind that you probably shouldn't attempt to enter a real race until

Signs you may have the bike racer mutation

- You draft strangers.

- You use a cycling social networking app that assigns you and other strangers an imaginary ranking that means nothing.

- You sprint whenever you pass those electronic road signs that tell you how fast you're going.

- You came across a professional bike race on TV once and actually watched it (as opposed to falling asleep, which is the normal reaction).

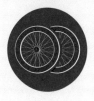

- You have purchased a piece of cycling equipment you don't need in the hopes that it will make you faster.

someone who is an actual bike racer tells you, "Hey, you should try racing."

If you go into it undercooked, you're liable to either get dropped immediately or crash everybody, or both.

TYPES OF RACING
Sanctioned

Your country has a national governing body (USA Cycling here) that sanctions bicycle competition. For a fee (get used to the fees), they will issue you something called a "racing license." Note that you *don't need to know how to race in order to obtain a license.* Nevertheless, this license will allow you to participate in organized cycling competitions across the typically recognized disciplines: road, track, mountain bike, cyclocross, and BMX.

ROAD

A road race can be anything from a stage race that lasts a week and covers an entire state, to something called a "criterium," wherein you ride around the block in some hick town for an hour.

Road racing is a good starting point for all kinds of bike racing, because after a while it will give you the strength and stamina (though probably not the bike-handling skills) you need to participate in the other disciplines as well.

TRACK

Like a criterium, track racing involves going around and around in a circle, only instead, you do it on a closed track called a "velodrome." As track racing enthusiasts will delight in telling you until you remind them to shut up, track racing was once the most popular sport in the United States, and there were velodromes everywhere. Sadly, this hasn't been the case for at least a hundred years, and velodromes have since gone the way of domestic manufacturing and phone booths: They still exist, but they're pretty rare. Therefore, depending on where you live, track racing may or may not be a viable option.

Track racing can be more fun than road racing, because instead of one big long race, it's a series of short races with different formats—kind of like a child's birthday party, only everyone takes themselves really seriously.

MOUNTAIN BIKE

Mountain bike racing can be an attractive proposition for the novice racer. In road racing, the pack dynamic forms the basis of the discipline, so if you find yourself getting dropped, there's little reason to continue. In mountain bike racing this dynamic is far less important, and even if you find yourself alone, there's still the challenge presented by the terrain. Plus, even if you're well off the lead, you will often find yourself engaged in a "race within a race" against another rider. Sure, you may be racing each other for thirtieth place, but glory is relative.

Another advantage of mountain bike racing for the novice is that when you crash you're not going to take fifty other riders down with you. Usually it's just one or two, and they have to scramble back out of the ravine before they can attempt to punch you.

CYCLOCROSS

Cyclocross is the fastest-growing discipline in terms of popularity. This is because riding around in a muddy field for forty-five minutes to an hour is an attractive proposition for competitors and spectators alike. For the competitor, there's no getting dropped and there's no getting lost. For the spectator, there's the advantage of actually being able to watch the races because the riders don't disappear down the road or into the woods. It's also pretty much the only type of bicycle race your noncycling friends or family members might humor you by attending, since the venues are often in some bucolic area, there's usually food and drink, and most people can deal with enjoying a seasonal beer in the fall.

BMX

BMX is the most family-friendly discipline and by far the most conducive to child participation and, therefore, an ideal choice for those cyclists who are fortunate enough to discover their BR+ status during their youth.

Nonsanctioned
GRASSROOTS RACING

In certain regions there are alternative organizations that form competition outside of the auspices of the national governing body. This frees them from the onerous financial and legal burdens imposed on participants and promoters by said national governing body. If you live in a hotbed of bicycle culture and do not labor under the delusion that you will one day become a professional, then grassroots racing presents an appealing option.

CLUBS

Technically you don't even need to know how to ride a bike in order to get a racing license. Therefore, before attempting a sanctioned bicycle race, you can learn the fundamentals of competition by joining a bicycle racing club. Clubs offer skills clinics, organized training rides, and sometimes even races just for members. Also, despite the independent nature of cycling, bike racing is fundamentally a team sport—indeed, in this sense, bike racing is a team sport for introverts. Therefore, riding with a club will teach you how the team dynamic works in cycling and allow you to meet fellow riders who could one day become your teammates.

UNDERGROUND

You don't need permission from an organization to have a bike race; all you need are two or more cyclists who want to see who's faster. Consequently, there are all kinds of unsanctioned and underground races. Some of these races are grimy and beer soaked, and others are buffed to a high sheen, packaged, sponsored, and chronicled extensively in the media. Examples include:

• **ALLEY CATS.** These used to be races for bike messengers that were designed to replicate their working conditions. Over the years they've become extremely popular and are now mostly scavenger hunts for millennials.

- **FIXED-GEAR CRITS.** People like to go fast on track bikes. However, there aren't that many velodromes, and if your goal is pure speed you may not be excited by the idea of participating in a contrived scavenger hunt for millennials. Given this, someone had a bright idea: "Hey, why don't we just race our track bikes around in circles on the street?" Thus the fixed-gear crit was born.
- **GRAVEL RACING.** It's exactly what it sounds like. The fields of flyover country are crisscrossed with gravel roads. People race bikes on them.
- **BIKEPACKING RACING.** Like gravel racing, only you go farther, carry luggage, and sleep along the way.

GRAN FONDOS

Gran fondos are based on the European model of taking thousands of road cyclists and unleashing them upon the countryside. At the front of the pack are some pros who have been fired from their teams for doping, and behind them is pretty much the entire spectrum of roadiedom.

Increasingly, this model is being imported to North America, where it's proven very popular. Riders love it because they're timed and get to measure their performance, yet at the same time it's nearly impossible to get dropped, owing to the vast size of the field. Promoters love it because thousands of riders means many thousands of dollars in entry fees, and if there's one thing true about roadies, it's that they'll pay almost anything to participate in an event that includes some kind of custom-designed jersey.

Branded gran fondos are also a reliable revenue stream for retired pros, who might otherwise be reduced to opening bike shops, starting coaching services, or doing sleep-inducing commentary during Tour de France broadcasts.

FINANCIAL IMPACT OF RACING

The financial impact of bike racing can be devastating.

On the face of it, bike racing may seem like an inexpensive proposition. After all, you've already got the bike, so all you really need to pay for is the license and the entry fee.

However, this fails to take into account the psychoactive component of bike racing, and that first race produces a change in the brain chemistry and function of the BR+ cyclist. There are many possible outcomes of your first race, but they all result in the same behavior:

• **Possible outcome #1: You win.** You are elated. Clearly you have a future in this sport. You resolve to upgrade your equipment immediately.

• **Possible outcome #2: You crash.** You are dejected. Clearly you have to correct the situation next time. In the meantime, you broke a bunch of stuff and ripped your shorts. You resolve to replace your equipment immediately.

• **Possible outcome #3: You get dropped.** You are dejected. Clearly you have to correct the situation next time. In the meantime, you read about some expensive wheels that are really fast. You resolve to buy a pair immediately.

• **Possible outcome #4: You finish somewhere in the middle.** You finished your first race without getting dropped. You are elated. It's only a matter of time before you're winning. You resolve to upgrade your equipment immediately.

And it doesn't stop there. Soon you'll travel to races. You'll need to pay for transportation and lodging. If you don't have a car, you'll want to get one; if you do, you'll want to outfit it with racks and accessories.

Then there's all the stuff you'll need for fitness:

— A stationary trainer

— Rollers

— Energy foods

— Energy drinks

— Recovery foods

— Recovery drinks

— Power meters and other data measurement systems

— Various lotions, embrocations, crotchal salves, and so forth

And don't forget the equipment! Even if you race only one discipline and have only one bike you'll still need multiple pairs of wheels with different gearing, various tires, every possible clothing permutation for every conceivable weather condition. Plus, you'll be piling on those miles, which means your equipment will wear out quickly—and that's if you're lucky enough not to crash, because thanks to today's brittle race bikes, a single spill can cost you thousands of dollars.

All of this is to say nothing about the coach you'll invariably consider hiring.

On the other hand, the only income you can expect to see is the odd $20 for finishing in third place—but you'll have to use that to buy your teammates waffles.

I know what you're thinking: "I don't *need* to buy into all that, do I? I can just 'run what I brung,' right?"

Yes, you can! But you won't. That's not how it works.

PHYSICAL IMPACT OF BIKE RACING

So you'll be poor, but at least you'll be in the greatest shape of your life, right?

Not exactly.

Yes, when you immerse yourself in the world of bike racing you do get really fit. Unfortunately, you're fit to do only one thing, which is ride a bike. This means, you turn from a human being into a pair of legs and an aerobic system, and the rest of your body (including your brain) wastes away, which basically makes you a frog.

Frogs are full of power and grace when using their legs to propel them through the water or launch themselves off a lily pad, but the rest of the time they're just goofy and awkward looking, and they're not the brightest creatures in the pond either.

That will be you.

You also won't feel too hot. Greg LeMond famously said, "It never gets easier; you just go faster." This is one hundred percent true—and off the bike it's even worse. Your body will hurt when you're not riding. That enviably aero flat-backed riding position you've acquired will make standing erect painful. Your legs will be sore, which means you'll dread staircases, and you'll find yourself constantly missing buses and trains because, yeah, like hell you're going to run for them. Depending on your complexion, you may also develop a conspicuous cyclist's tan, which is really just a euphemism for a farmer's tan, and while other BR+ people may admire your new color scheme as a sign of your dedication, you'll mostly just look funny at the beach.

LIFESTYLE IMPACT OF BIKE RACING

While your cycling tan may make you look funny at the beach, that doesn't really matter, because you'll probably never go to the beach again.

In fact, there's a lot of fun stuff you won't do anymore, because now you're a bike racer.

Forget winning. Simply maintaining the cycling fitness necessary to hang with the pack requires lots and lots of riding. This means that if you tally up the hours you spend "training," you're easily giving up one whole day a week in service to bike racing—and that doesn't even include the racing itself.

Imagine losing an entire day of your life every single week!

It's like being an alcoholic, only a lot more expensive.

That lost day's going to have to come from somewhere, and if you have a job, this means you'll need to poach it from your leisure time. This seems harmless enough at first. So you give up knitting, pickling, binge watching TV shows, or whatever else you used to do on your own time.

Big deal.

However, it's easy to forget that your leisure time is also when you enjoy life with friends, family, and loved ones—all of whom will soon get used to a state of constant disappointment when you vanish into the horizon on yet another six-hour ride instead of going to the playground or visiting the farmer's market or simply holding hands and staring into each other's eyes.

Oh, sure, you'll go on a date that evening, but when your partner looks into your eyes all he'll see is a hollow, wasted shell, because you'll be tired and gutted after yet another "epic" day in the saddle.

Of course, there's always the possibility that your partner will also be a bike racer. Not only is this relatively rare, but it's also exponentially more unhealthy, because odds are you'll wind up just like Sid and Nancy—scrawny, broke, and strung out on bikes.

FINDING A BALANCE

All of the above notwithstanding, it is still possible to lead a productive life as a BR+ individual by taking the following steps:

• **Commute by bike.** Bike racers tend to think any ride that doesn't involve getting dressed up in special clothes doesn't count, but this isn't the case, and in fact every pedal stroke makes you stronger—even if it's on a Citi Bike. (Actually, *especially* if it's a Citi Bike, given that they weigh fifty pounds.)

So instead of carving hours out of your day just for training, integrate cycling into the more mundane areas of life and build fitness while getting things done.

• **Diversify.** Instead of obsessing over one racing discipline, take the ecumenical approach and dabble in all of them. Obsessing over one type of cycling can make you humorless and miserable, and nobody likes to be around humorless and miserable people. (Well, except roadies.)

• **Practice humility.** One of the most dangerous aspects of bike racing is that the amateur is only one or two degrees of separation from the professional. Indeed, if you're a midcategory racer, it's conceivable you might find yourself in the same race as a professional—or at least people who race against professionals— on a fairly regular basis.

The problem with this is that you might fall victim to the delusion that you could become a pro too. There are two problems with this:

1. You're not going to become a pro.

2. Even if you were capable of becoming a pro, you don't want to. In terms of success, the best-case scenario for a pro cyclist is Lance Armstrong, and nobody in their right mind would aspire to that.

Therefore, it's important to keep your own abilities in perspective, and to that end, you should remind yourself of the following on a regular basis:

You suck!

It sounds cruel, but it's actually the kindest thing you can say to yourself, because instead of allowing your hobby to crush you under the weight of your own aspirations, you can stop taking it all so seriously and start having fun.

Chapter 9

CYCLING WITH KIDS

You're a cyclist now and you love it!

In fact, you love it so much you're ready to pass your knowledge and excitement along to the next generation.

Good for you. There is no gift you can give a child that is greater than the gift of cycling—except for love, and shelter, and sustenance, and education, and health care.

But that's not all. When you introduce a child to bikes, you are also giving a gift to the entire cycling world, for when children grow up thinking cycling is normal, then we, as a society, get that much closer to a future in which it actually is.

Cue the Whitney Houston.

SOCIAL MORES AND JUDGMENT

On one hand, many people think bikes are for kids, and that when you get older you should drive a car.

On the other hand, fewer kids are actually riding bikes today. In fact, according to the organization Safe Routes to School, in 1969, forty-eight percent of kindergarten through eighth grade students walked or rode a bike to school.

By 2009, that number was down to fifteen percent, with forty-five percent arriving by "personal vehicle."

It's a sad state of affairs. We want our children to be healthy

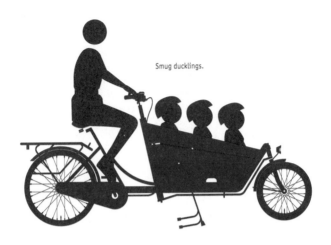

Smug ducklings.

and fit. At the same time, we want them to be safe. So instead of letting them ride their bikes, we shuttle them to school in our SUVs—which makes sense, because we need to protect them from all the other SUVs.

This safety-first mentality now extends to the actual riding of bikes—and scooters, and roller skates, and tricycles, and pretty much every wheeled means of conveyance for juveniles. Go visit a playground. (With your kid, of course. Don't go alone or you'll get arrested.) Notice how many children wear helmets, elbow pads, and kneepads while they're wheeling around, stiff and stilted like the Tin Man or a Storm Trooper from *Star Wars*.

When we treat riding a bike as something that requires donning maximum safety gear at all times, the prospect of riding bikes becomes about as appealing to a kid as going to the dentist.

Carrying your child on your bike as a passenger can also raise eyebrows. Plenty of people do this in the park or on the multi-use path. But if you actually use your bike as a means of family transport around town, prepare to become a local curiosity. Some will find it charming. Some will silently judge you. And some will not-so-silently judge you and vilify you openly for risking your child's safety.

But your children are never really safe in transit, thanks mostly to cars. The family minivan is not the safe haven the commercials make it out to be. Statistically speaking, the leading cause of injury-related death for children by a significant margin is riding in automobiles. So as long as you approach cycling with your child with due caution, you're certainly not exposing them to undue risk. You know exactly where they are, and you're rarely going more than fifteen miles per hour.

It's too bad we've become so repressed when it comes to bikes. For kids, the bike is their first taste of self-directed, independent transport, and riding a bike exercises the body as well as the mind. For adults, transporting your kid by bike introduces a whole new dimension of fun and practicality to everyday life, and it can be a respite from the hassle of looking for parking and sitting in traffic.

CARRYING YOUR CHILD ON THE BIKE

The key to making sure your child is comfortable traveling by bicycle is to start them young. Check your local laws concerning how old a child must be to be carried on a bicycle, then use your judgment. In New York City, the rule is one year. This is a pretty good guideline. Children should be able to sit up straight for prolonged periods of time, with good muscular control of their great big baby heads.

Speaking of that great big baby head, you should put a helmet on it, at least to begin with. First, it's almost certainly the law where

Is your child ready to ride on a bike?

1. Put baby on floor in seated position
2. Approach baby
3. Gently push baby
4. If baby stays upright and giggles, baby is ready
5. If baby falls over and cries, wait two weeks and repeat

you live. Second, if your child is going to fall off the bike, it's much more likely to be the result of the bike falling over while you're mounting or dismounting than because of a crash out on the road. So the helmet is a hedge against such mishaps.

Of course, in addition to a child, you'll also need a child seat for your bike. Some mount to your bike in the front and some mount in the rear. There are advantages and disadvantages to each.

Options for Child Seats
FRONTAL BABY POSITIONING

There are various styles of front child seats. The most common ones clamp to your steer tube between your stem and headset so the bike handles relatively normally and you've got room to operate the controls. They're fairly simple to install and most are designed to be easily removable when you're not using them, but if you're unsure of compatibility with your bike you should consult your bike shop.

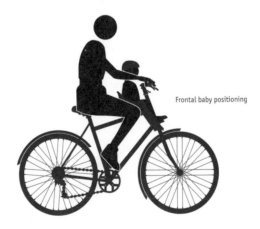

Frontal baby positioning

✔ ADVANTAGES
— Like dogs, children love putting their faces in the wind.
— You can see and interact with your child while riding (fun subjects of discussion include Elmo, fart sounds, and other vital issues of the day).

— As with inanimate loads, bikes handle a bit more naturally and comfortably when loaded in front.

✗ DISADVANTAGES

— May be a bit awkward with larger children.

REAR BABY POSITIONING

Rear child seats usually clamp to your frame or to your rear rack, and some include quick-release brackets that let you switch the seat between different bicycles. Consult the helpful, courteous professionals at your local bike shop.

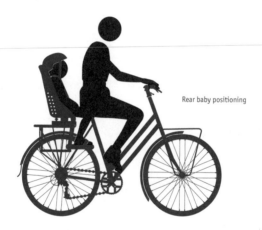

Rear baby positioning

✔ ADVANTAGES

— May be more suitable for your larger child.
— You don't have to interact with your child if you don't want to. ("Will you stop it with the fart sounds?!?")
— More head support, so may be easier for your child to nap on longer rides.

✗ DISADVANTAGES

— Mounting and dismounting is a bit trickier, and if you're not careful you could karate kick baby in face.

— Conversations are difficult, and you'll both be shouting "What? What?" at each other like an elderly couple at dinner.

As an alternative to child seats, you might also consider a bike trailer.

BIKE TRAILER

Child bike trailers usually look like jogging strollers—in fact, you can even get combination stroller/bike trailers. Bike trailers usually clamp to your rear chainstay and they roll on pneumatic tires.

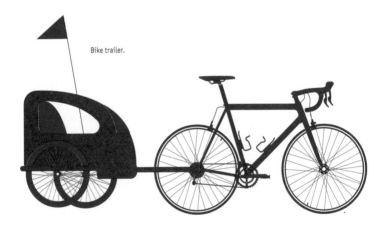

Bike trailer.

✔ ADVANTAGES

— You can fit a bike trailer to all sorts of bikes that might otherwise not easily accommodate a child seat, such as your road bike or your mountain bike.
— You can carry two children at a time, and since they're enclosed, kids are that much less likely to drop their toys in the middle of the road.
— If the trailer is convertible to a stroller, you can keep on rolling them when you get off the bike.
— Kids love being inside small, claustrophobic, pet-carrier-like spaces.
— When not carrying children, you can use it to carry beer.

✗ DISADVANTAGES

— Difficult to store when not in use.

— Large size may be awkward in some riding situations.

— Trailer is low and may not be visible to other road users.

GETTING STARTED RIDING WITH YOUR CHILD

Once you've set up your child bike seat or trailer, the first thing to remember is that your bike handles differently when it is loaded with baby weight. If you've been carrying groceries or camping supplies you already know this, but if you haven't, you should take some time to get used to the difference. Take extra care when mounting or dismounting the bike, because the bike can very easily tip over, even if it's equipped with a kickstand. (For maximum stability, you might want to consider a centerstand if your bike will accept one.)

Your bike isn't the only thing that will feel different; you'll feel a

Cargo bikes

Most kids outgrow their bike seats by about four years or so, but by this time your family will probably have become bike dependent to at least some degree, which means you'll still want to be able to carry the kid around town.

But how?

At this point in their lives, children are becoming "active passengers." They can get on and off your bike themselves. They can hold on. They don't need to be restrained with straps.

Therefore, if you're serious about kid-schlepping by bike, you'll want to get some kind of cargo bike or Dutch bike. This will allow for a "hop-on, hop-off" setup as opposed to a molded plastic seat, and you'll be able to carry your child at least until they're old enough to hate you and refuse to be seen with you.

Another advantage of the cargo bike is that some will allow you to carry both your child *and* your child's bike. This is great when you're teaching your kid to ride, because if they get tired or frustrated you can always just load up the bike and the kid and head straight to the ice cream shop.

lot different too. After all, this is your child, so at first you'll experience a sense of extreme hyper-alertness. "Slow down, you maniac!" you'll be tempted to yell at that elderly person on the Rascal.

Don't worry, it will all start to feel normal soon enough.

Start out with short trips to the playground, the park, or the local shops before attempting anything ambitious in order to build your child's on-the-bike stamina. You don't want the kid melting down when you're an hour from home.

TEACHING YOUR CHILD TO RIDE
When to Start

Parents obsess over milestones. "Is she walking? Is she talking? Is she potty trained?"

It's all meaningless. We're all walking and talking and using the toilet now—sometimes all at once. So what's the difference when we started? It's not like we brag about when we were potty trained at cocktail parties.

The same goes for riding bikes. How old your child is when you start teaching them to ride depends on both you and the child. Show the kid a balance bike. Are they interested? Are they able to straddle it? If the answer to both of these questions is yes, then let 'er rip.

If they start crying, put it in the closet and wait until they ask for it.

Which Method?

Traditionally, in North America at least, children learn to ride on a bike with training wheels. The training wheels keep the bike upright. As the kid gets used to the bike, you raise the training wheels incrementally until the child begins to balance the bike a bit on their own. Then, once they seem like they know what they're doing, you take the training wheels off and ta-da!

The kid falls over.

Today, instead of the training-wheel method, balance bikes are becoming more and more popular. Balance bikes are basically just bikes without pedals that the child pushes along like he's Fred Flintstone. The idea is that your child first learns to balance by riding the balance bike, and then once they master that, they're able to hop onto a regular bike and pedal happily away into the horizon.

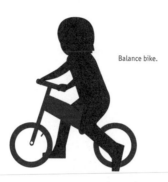

Balance bike.

Consequently there's been a bit of a backlash against training wheels, especially among the more progressive types of cycling parents who shop at food co-ops. This is because training wheels are hopelessly American, whereas balance bikes are excitingly European.

There is something to this shift. After all, training wheels don't allow a bicycle to lean, and leaning is how you keep a bike upright. So how is a child supposed to learn anything when they're essentially riding a tricycle?

The balance bike, on the other hand, teaches the child the *physics* of the bicycle, which is arguably the hardest and most important aspect to master. Plus, they're easy to ride and lots of fun.

But even though training wheels are now considered deeply uncool and pathetically Victorian, don't count them out, because they are still very useful for teaching your child to pedal (as well as to brake).

For this reason, you may want to supply your child with both a balance bike *and* a regular bike with training wheels and let them go back and forth as they see fit. More than anything, fun is what's going to encourage them to learn, so when it's time to ride, you should let them choose the one that's going to give them the most enjoyment at that moment.

This way, they can master the balancing and the pedaling in a parallel fashion, and then combine the two when they're good and ready.

What Kind of Bike?

There are sporty balance bikes with handbrakes, and there are simple balance bikes made of wood.

Get whichever's cheapest.

It's just a seat and some wheels. Don't overthink it.

In fact, you don't even need a balance bike. If you're handy you can just use a regular bike and remove the cranks and chain, then put them back on again when the time comes.

There are also various companies that make fancy kids' bikes. They will explain to you how their bikes are ergonomically designed with children's unique proportions in mind. They'll also explain that riding an awesome bike now will ensure your child loves riding forever, whereas if they ride a bike from a department store they'll be scarred for life.

Come on.

Clearly you don't want to put your kid on a rusty hulk with sharp edges that will give them tetanus, but beyond that, you don't need to be too picky. Keep in mind that your kid will outgrow this thing in a matter of months anyway. By buying your kid a fancy bike you're really just projecting your own bike-weenie desires onto them—which is fine, but certainly not necessary.

If you can find a hand-me-down kid's bike for free, then that's great. They're all over the place, in basements and garages all across the country. Or if you need or want to get something new, go to the bike shop you love and buy a bike from them. All the bike companies offer inexpensive kids' bikes, and the shop will no doubt have some useful tips for you as well.

Plus, picking out some accessories (a horn, a bell, a helmet) will make the prospect that much more exciting for your child.

Chances are your kid will outgrow the bike before the tires wear out, but if you want to amortize the purchase you can always have more kids.

Bike Setup

Speaking of projecting your own bike weeniedom onto your kid, when setting up the bike, don't apply your weeniesh adult bike fit standards. Don't worry about optimal leg extension and maximum power transfer. Ignore the doofus on Facebook who says your kid's saddle is too low. The most important goal when setting up your child's bike is that they feel confident when riding. They should be able to flat-foot the bike and reach the handlebar grips without having to lean forward. This will allow them to master the bike. The rest is irrelevant. You can start fine-tuning the bike for maximum efficiency in about five years.

When Are They Ready?

When your kid is carving corners on the balance bike and laying down skids on the pedal bike it's time to lose the balance bike and the training wheels and fly solo.

They may be two, or they may be six. It doesn't really matter.

It's possible your child may indeed ride off into the horizon right away, but if they don't, the best place to start is a grassy surface with a slight incline. Riding down the incline will make it easy for the child to build the necessary momentum to stay upright, and the grass will mitigate the inevitable fall.

Repeat this until they figure it out or get flustered, whichever comes first.

If they do get flustered, just try again later. It won't be long before your child figures it out and you're both jumping up and down with glee.

Helmet or No Helmet?

Laws aside, the health benefits of cycling for children far outweigh the risks. Also, keep in mind that your young child will be riding a bike with a teeny-tiny gear. This means they almost certainly won't be able to ride any faster than they run—unless you send them down a mountain road, which you're not going to do. So try to keep the level of "danger" in perspective.

Pick a safe spot to ride—that's by far the most important.

A lot of kids *want* to wear helmets, since if there's one thing that's true about children it's that they like to put funny-looking stuff on their heads.

Ultimately you should do what makes both you and your child the happiest. If the helmet makes them feel like a racer, then great. If they hate it, then skip it. If they don't care either way, then just do what makes you most comfortable.

BEING A ROLE MODEL FOR YOUR CHILD

One of the hardest parts of being a parent is keeping track of all the stuff you're going to have to reteach them later on:

"Santa lives in the North Pole."

"Mommy and Daddy weren't fighting. We were having a discussion."

"Your goldfish has to go back to the ocean now." (Cue flushing sound.)

For now it's best to keep things simple, but in a few years you're going to have to have a little talk.

Your child is also going to come home with some funny ideas about bikes, since the automotive industrial complex starts brainwashing at an early age. For example, when they start learning about vehicles in preschool, guess which one never makes the list. (Hint: It has two wheels, pedals, and smug people ride them to Whole Foods.)

It's important to teach your child that bicycles are normal. You don't want to be a gigantic doofus about it, but you also want to counteract any brainwashing before it festers. ("No, Sally, your teacher is wrong. Bikes *do* belong on the road.") Most of this will probably happen as a natural consequence of your being a cyclist, but nevertheless it's something to keep in mind.

This also extends to the way you ride. When you're on the bike, try to keep your cool. Sure, the driver who just cut you off may technically qualify as an ass clown, but that doesn't mean you should call him one while your kid's sitting behind you.

At the same time, the vantage point of the bicycle affords you a good opportunity to educate your child about the workings of the road, and you'll be able to point things out that they'd never see from the backseat of a minivan. It's also an opportunity to show them how courteous you are to pedestrians (which you *always* are, right?), since you're not separated from them by a pane of shatter-proof glass.

Then there's the bicycle itself. "How does the bike go?" "Which one's the brake?" "What does this lever do?" Show them. Let them help you pump up the tires. Plus, by being a passenger, your child will come to feel at home on the bike and will probably learn to ride that much easier themselves.

And don't forget navigation! Riding with your child will enhance their understanding of their neighborhood, and they'll be that much more equipped to get around by themselves when the time comes.

Try not to be too smug about it, but also savor the fact that, by growing up on and around bicycles, your child will experience something too many others miss out on—and whether they grow up to be cyclists or not really doesn't matter.

(As long as they don't become roadies.)

Chapter 10

WHAT THE FUTURE HOLDS

The year is 2315. The ice caps have melted. The seas have risen hundreds of feet, inundating the great cities of the world. The one percent has hoarded the last of the fossil fuels to power their sump pumps and Jacuzzis, while the rest of us pedal around on bamboo paddleboats and toil for meager wages at massive desalination plants and retail centers.

Yeah, I know, you don't care about the *distant* future. You're worried about your own lifetime, and maybe that of your kids if you have them. Specifically, you want to know if this whole bike thing is a good long-term investment.

It is.

The jury is still out on what's going to become of humanity and the planet, but pending our demise, the future of cycling is so bright it's hard to look directly at it without squinting. Consider the fact that for most of the last century the automobile did its best to literally and figuratively kill the bicycle. It failed. Indeed, cycling is more robust than ever. The bicycle remains the most ubiquitous vehicle on the planet. Cities are continuing to install more and more bicycle infrastructure. And roadies, in the throes of weeniedom, are willing to spend up to $20,000 on the latest carbon superbike.

You can't say any of that about Rollerblades.

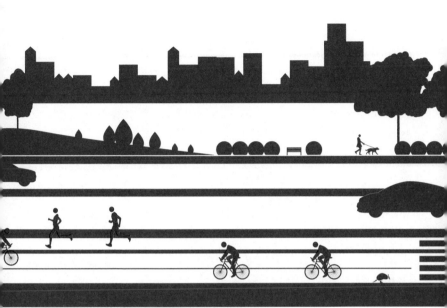

This isn't to say cycling won't continue to experience its ups and downs. Since the days of the penny farthing, cyclists have been beset by political opposition, vehicular intimidation, and marketing gimmickry. This will never change.

Nevertheless, as long as cycling remembers its past, it will ride triumphantly into the future, even in an ever-changing transportation landscape.

INFRASTRUCTURE

Many cities have made unprecedented investments in bike lanes and other amenities (necessities, really), and this will continue. Depending on where you live, cycling infrastructure growth may slow down occasionally as politicians pander to shortsighted people who don't see the value of a bike infrastructure.

They'll come around. They'll *have* to come around, because the simple fact is that there are too many cars! It's not even a moral issue so much as a spatial one. The number of registered motor vehicles on the road in the United States alone increases by well over three million a year, and this has been the case since 1960. Meanwhile, our antiquated car-centric infrastructure is crumbling. Bridges are collapsing. Highways are riddled with potholes. Eventually we're going to run out of roads to drive our cars on and fuel to put in them and places to store them when we're not using them.

Of course, we won't abandon the car. Why would we? Humankind simply does not walk away from that level of convenience, and we'll keep figuring out ways to refine them and keep them in our lives. However, at the same time, and in cities especially, transportation will certainly become more nuanced and multifaceted, and bikes will continue to be a significant part of this transformation. There's no more efficient vehicle for short distance travel in a densely populated environment, and as we refine the infrastructure to accommodate bicycles, more and more people will incorporate them into their everyday lives.

And none of this even takes into account the sheer pleasure you get from riding a bike. This has been true since the days of the penny farthing, and even before when people puttered about on dandy horses. Cycling appeals to people so deeply and fulfills such a basic kinetic human desire that it's almost like the bicycle is a classic element for life: earth, water, fire, air, and bikes. We'll probably be riding the things until humanity becomes extinct or we upload ourselves to some digitized mass consciousness and the planet is consumed in flames.

So in the (near) future, expect more bike lane ribbon-cutting ceremonies as giant iron girders fall off the bridge in the background.

SELF-DRIVING CARS

Automobiles attacked hard during the last century, and bikes successfully managed to fight them off. Since then, there's been a shift in the popular consciousness as more and more people are waking up to the fact that cars are big, dangerous, environmentally unfriendly, and obnoxious.

Still, we cannot afford to become complacent.

Cars will never surrender their fight for control of the roads, but they will change their tactics for the twenty-first century to something more cunning.

Back in the day, cars were intimidating behemoths. They were big. They guzzled gas audibly. They had razor-sharp tailfins or shiny chrome bumpers or gleaming grilles. When you saw one, you coveted it immediately, to the point where you were ready to take out a second mortgage in order to own one. At the same time, you knew to get the hell out of its way before it ate you like the Plymouth Fury in *Christine*.

Cars ruled by instilling both awe and fear.

Now that we've arrived in the twenty-first century, we have a different attitude toward cars. These are kinder, gentler, more artisanal times. Instead of a car that frightens us, we're looking for a car that wants to be our friend—like an iPhone or a roomie.

Hence the self-driving car.

It's hard to object to a technology that promises to make the road a safer place. At the same time, at this point in history, trusting cars is like trusting that cheating ex-boyfriend who insists he's changed for good this time. Are you really going to take him back? It's all a bit too good to be true.

The best-case scenario for the self-driving car is that drivers become obsolete, road rage vanishes from the face of the planet, and we all share the roads in safety and bliss, exchanging flowers and chocolates at intersections.

Hey, it could happen.

The worst-case scenario is that, once we eliminate the human factor from driving, any car-bike mishap will *always* be the cyclist's fault.

When it's your word against the computer, who do you think they're going to believe?

Consider also the extent to which drivers have successfully shifted the onus of safety onto every other road user. Wear your helmet. Wear reflective clothing. And when the driver hits you anyway, "The cyclist came out of nowhere" is considered a perfectly acceptable excuse.

So what happens in a few years or a few decades when you're sharing the road with an operating system instead of a driver? We're already seeing glimpses. For example, Volvo recently displayed a "connected car and helmet prototype" so that drivers and cyclists can avoid crashing into each other. Basically, your helmet alerts you to the presence of a Volvo, and the Volvo alerts its driver to the presence of a cyclist wearing a Volvo-detecting helmet. On the surface, it's an added layer of safety. What's the big deal? But what happens if (or probably when) self-driving cars take over? Will these "connected helmets" become mandatory? Will cyclists be required to wear homing beacons? By 2025, will you be inserting a connected suppository before every ride?

One of the most appealing aspects of cycling is its accessibility. All you need to do is throw a leg over and go. Electronic encumbrances could compromise this accessibility just as mandatory helmet laws compromise it today.

THE BIKE OF THE FUTURE

Electronic shifting systems . . . integrated turn signals . . . smart locks . . .

Whatever.

Fundamentally there's not much difference between your bike and the safety bicycles of the late nineteenth century, save for some admittedly neat refinements. These refinements will, of course, continue to evolve, but in the meantime you don't need to worry about any of them until it's time to buy a new bike, at which point your next bike will have them and you'll appreciate them for about two hours until you start to take them for granted.

In the meantime, thanks to crowdsourced funding, would-be entrepreneurs will attempt to revolutionize the bicycle in various ways, mostly by integrating it with your smartphone. However, they're not revolutionizing the bike so much as they're merely "niftifying" it. Sure, a bike with handlebar grips that vibrate when it's time to turn is nifty, but when you consider that you're rarely riding more than a dozen miles from your home anyway, who really cares?

It's all just more stuff to plug in.

Notification aside, the two biggies in terms of bike innovation in the twenty-first century will most likely turn out to be:

1. Bike share. Electronic helmets probably aren't going to change the face of cycling, but electronic networks of publicly available bicycles certainly will. In fact, they're doing it already. Bike share systems (Citi Bike in New York being the obvious example) are increasingly commonplace, and they'll continue to become indispensable fixtures in cities and towns everywhere. You'll simply come to expect them, like hotel cable or free Wi-Fi in a café. Bike share closes gaps in public transit and splits the difference between driving and walking in dense areas. Perhaps just as important, bike share elevates cycling to a level of accessibility and ubiquity that helps legitimize and normalize it.

2. E-bikes. Bicycles with electric motor assists have the potential to make various forms of everyday, practical cycling accessible and attractive to a whole new demographic. Consider carrying stuff. The idea of hauling groceries and kids by bike is daunting enough to the layperson, and if you throw a few hills in there, the prospect is completely off the table. Add a motor into the equation though and suddenly the bike as family SUV becomes possible, or maybe even attractive. The same thing goes for commuting in hot weather, since a few watts of assistance might mean the difference between sweating through your clothes and arriving to the office as dry as a piece of Melba toast.

The downside is that as e-bikes become more common, you might have to dodge e-assisted riders on the mountain bike trail or on the sidewalk. This can be solved with a phone app that emits an electromagnetic pulse and disables the motor. Look for one on Kickstarter.

GETTING OLD

So what about you?

Well, you'll be glad to know that cycling fights the aging process. Consider this: Researchers chose eighty-four males and forty-one females between the ages of fifty-five and seventy-nine, all of whom were fit cyclists. Then they tested their endurance, muscle mass, balance, bone density, and a bunch of other stuff. In all categories, the results showed they functioned like people much younger than their actual age.*

And yes, this is an actual study and not the plot of the 1985 science fiction movie *Cocoon.*

Not only does cycling keep you young, but you also won't have to give it up for golf because your body can't take it anymore. This is because cycling is a low-impact activity, whereas running will eventually pulverize your joints and you'll need a new hip—at which point you'll have to take up cycling anyway, so it's a good thing you're starting now.

Hey, worst case, you'll need a recumbent.

But we don't ride just for the health benefits, just as we don't drink wine just for the antioxidants.

You will have a lifelong relationship with cycling because riding a bike will help you make sense of both yourself and the world. The act of pedaling can help you untie those knotty problems or dissolve that ball of stress in your gut. (Not to mention reduce the size of your actual gut.) You'll discover new places, and you'll come

---

* No word on whether they were wearing helmets.

to appreciate the familiar ones more deeply. If you're doing it right, as you get older, your equipment and riding style will change along with your body and your diminishing sense of urgency, but your love for it will remain the same. You'll always derive a sense of deep satisfaction from the act of cycling, and at the same time you'll find it endlessly compelling—as though this mysteriously balancing machine is an etching needle, and you're using it to trace the contours of some greater truth.

Now go out and ride your bike.

Index